小児科外来
Medical English for Pediatric Outpatients
医療英語

編集 **中村安秀** 大阪大学大学院人間科学研究科教授
中野貴司 川崎医科大学小児科教授

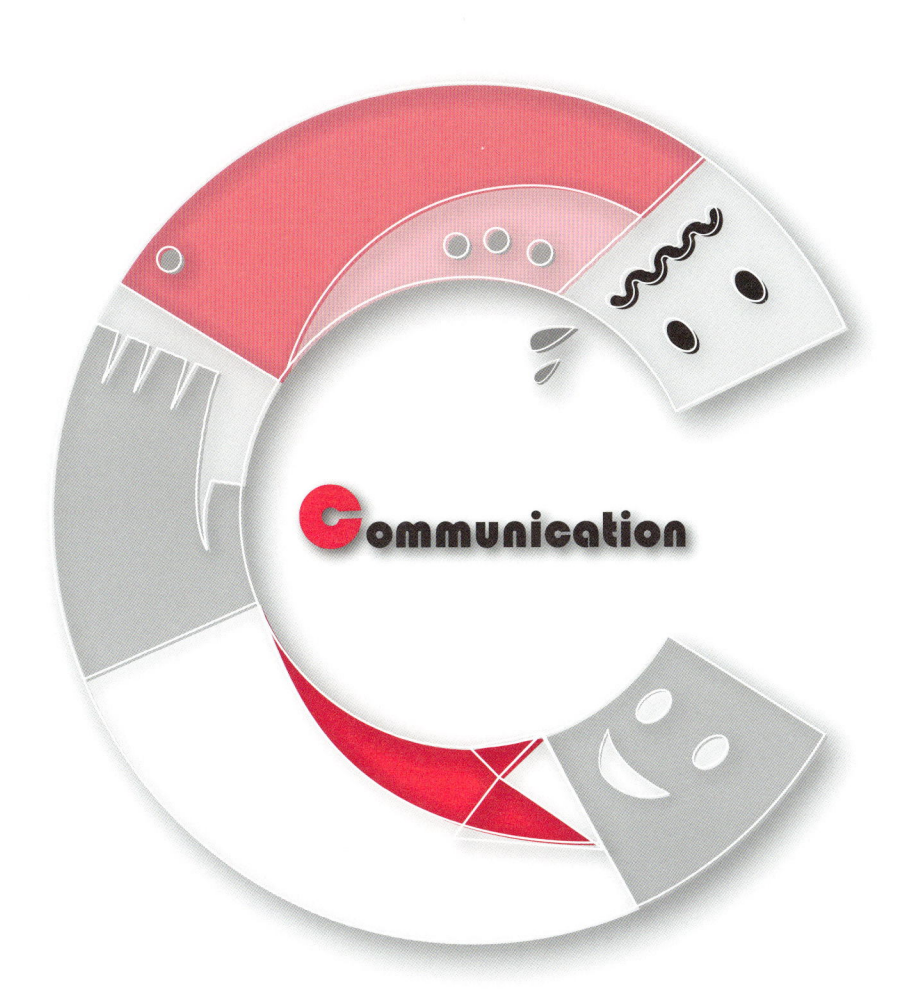

Communication

診断と治療社

序文

　私たちは，実は「小児科外来医療英語」という本を上梓するほど，英語は流暢ではありません．いまの若い世代の小児科医が話す滑らかな英語に聞きほれてしまうくらいです．

　ただ，ともに若輩の時代から，アジアやアフリカの地で，英語を使わなければ何ごとも始まらないという環境のなかで，必要に迫られて，英語で話す度胸だけは十分に鍛えられました．また，子どもの病気や健康状態を把握するためには，言葉だけでなく，その背後にある文化や習慣を理解しておくことの重要性も教えられました．

　いま，日本には多くの外国人が暮らしています．小児科の外来や入院病棟で，外国人の姿を見かけることはふつうのことになっています．できるだけ実践の場で役立つように，診断書や説明書の見本も掲載しました．この「小児科外来医療英語」というツールを使っていただき，自信を持って外国人の子どもや家族に話しかけてください．異国で病院にかかるというのは，不安なもの．医師や看護師のやさしい言葉や明るい笑顔が，信頼と安心の源です．少しくらい発音が違っていてもかまいません．「習うより慣れろ」の気持ちで，どうか，英語での診察を楽しんでいただけますように！

　なお，本書の英語については，プロフェッショナルな医療通訳士の皆さん方に執筆・翻訳をお願いしました．西野かおるさん，Cindy Roatさん，竹迫和美さん，ホワイトみどりさんには，この場を借りて厚く御礼申しあげます．

　小児科に特化した実践的な英語をめざしたつもりですが，他に類書がなく試行錯誤しながら手探りで編集作業をしてきました．まだまだ改善の余地はあるのではないかと思っています．読者の方から，忌憚ないご意見やご指摘をいただければ幸いです．

2011年12月

中村安秀　中野貴司

目次

第1章 / Part 1　診察をする前に：多文化診療入門
Before examine the foreign child
（中村安秀）

1　外国人の子どもを診察するということ ……………………………… 2

第2章 / Part 2　英語で子どもを診る：英語を使った小児科診療・総論
To examine the patient
（西野かおる/Cindy Roat）

1　あいさつ ……………………………………………………………… 10
2　症状を聞く …………………………………………………………… 14
3　既往歴を聞く ………………………………………………………… 19
4　診察する ……………………………………………………………… 22
5　検査をしましょう …………………………………………………… 26
6　診断を伝える ………………………………………………………… 30
7　薬の説明 ……………………………………………………………… 34
8　会計時のトラブルをさけるために ………………………………… 47

第3章 / Part 3　症状を英語で把握する：英語を使った小児科診療・各論
To understand the patient's symptom
（中村安秀）

1　基本的な問診 ………………………………………………………… 54
2　健診 …………………………………………………………………… 57
3　栄養方法 ……………………………………………………………… 62
4　先天性代謝異常症などの検査 ……………………………………… 64
5　よくみる症状 ………………………………………………………… 65

第4章 / Part 4　病気を英語で説明する：英語を使った小児科診療・病名編
To explain the patient's disease
（福島慎二）

1　かぜ症候群 …………………………………………………………… 68
2　インフルエンザ ……………………………………………………… 70
3　溶連菌感染症 ………………………………………………………… 72
4　肺炎 …………………………………………………………………… 74
5　急性中耳炎 …………………………………………………………… 76
6　急性胃腸炎 …………………………………………………………… 78
7　食中毒 ………………………………………………………………… 80
8　尿路感染症 …………………………………………………………… 82
9　突発性発疹 …………………………………………………………… 84
10　熱性けいれん ………………………………………………………… 86

（田中孝明）

11　手足口病 ･･ *88*
12　ヘルパンギーナ ･･････････････････････････････････ *90*
13　麻疹（はしか） ･･････････････････････････････････ *92*
14　風疹 ･･ *94*
15　おたふくかぜ ････････････････････････････････････ *96*
16　水ぼうそう ･･････････････････････････････････････ *98*
17　百日咳 ･･ *100*
18　川崎病 ･･ *102*
19　てんかん ･･ *104*
20　先天性心疾患 ････････････････････････････････････ *106*

（浅田和豊）

21　気管支ぜんそく ･･････････････････････････････････ *109*
22　アトピー性皮膚炎 ････････････････････････････････ *112*
23　食物アレルギー ･･････････････････････････････････ *115*
24　じんましん ･･････････････････････････････････････ *118*
25　糖尿病 ･･ *121*
26　肥満 ･･ *124*
27　外傷・打撲 ･･････････････････････････････････････ *127*
28　熱傷 ･･ *130*
29　誤飲・誤嚥 ･･････････････････････････････････････ *133*

第5章 Part 5　診断書・説明書編
Medical certificate・prescription

（中野貴司）

- 証明書テンプレートのダウンロードサービスについて ････ *138*
- 予防接種証明書　テンプレートダウンロード可 ････････････ *140*
- 健康診断書　テンプレートダウンロード可 ････････････････ *144*
- 診断書　テンプレートダウンロード可 ････････････････････ *145*
- 説明と同意書 ･･ *146*
- 通院証明書 ･･ *148*
- 入院証明書 ･･ *149*
- 入院診療計画書 ･･････････････････････････････････････ *150*
- 通園・登校許可書 ････････････････････････････････････ *152*
- 分娩予定日証明書 ････････････････････････････････････ *153*
- 分娩証明書 ･･ *154*

索引 ･･ *155*

執筆者一覧

編集・執筆者

中村安秀	大阪大学大学院人間科学研究科　教授
中野貴司	川崎医科大学小児科　教授

執筆者　（執筆順，敬称・肩書略）

西野かおる	神戸薬科大学英語非常勤講師・薬剤師
Cindy Roat	全米医療通訳コンサルタント
福島慎二	東京医科大学病院渡航者医療センター
田中孝明	川崎医科大学附属川崎病院小児科
浅田和豊	国立病院機構三重病院小児科

翻訳者／翻訳協力者

竹迫和美	IMIA 国際医療通訳士協会日本支部，大阪大学大学院人間科学研究科
ホワイトみどり	フリーランス医療通訳者，ミルトン整形外科・スポーツ理学療法プラクティスマネージャー

1章

診察をする前に
（多文化診療入門）

Before examine the foreign child

The aim of this chapter

在日外国人の人口推移や文化・言語の扱いの違いによるさまざまな問題，診療の際にとても役立つ海外の母子健康手帳について，知ることができます．

Part 1　1．診察をする前に：多文化診療入門

1　外国人の子どもを診察するということ

1．外国人の子どもが増えている！

　外国人登録者数は増加の一途をたどり，2009年末には約219万人で，総人口の約1.7％を占めています．外国人登録者の国籍数は190（無国籍も含む）．国籍別にみると，中国（31.1％），韓国・朝鮮（26.5％），ブラジル，フィリピン，ペルー，アメリカ合衆国と続いています．都道府県別には，外国人登録者数が最も多いのは東京都（約42万人）で，以下，愛知県，大阪府，神奈川県，埼玉県，千葉県，兵庫県，静岡県，茨城県，京都府の順となっています．大阪府では韓国・朝鮮が多く，東海地域ではブラジルやペルーが多いといったように，地域ごとに特徴があります．

　最近の外国人の人口動態の特徴は，外国人家族の定住傾向が明らかとなってきたことです．定住化に伴う最も大きな変化は，国際結婚の増加と外国人を親にもつ子どもの増加です．2006年には，婚姻総数約73万件のうち，国際結婚が4万4千件となり，婚姻総数の6.1％を占めています．とくに，夫が日本人で妻が外国人という国際結婚が増加しています．外国人妻の国籍をみると，中国，フィリピン，韓国・朝鮮，タイで約90％を占めています．国際結婚の増加にともない，外国人を親にもつ子どもも増加しています．2007年には，出生総数は109万人でしたが，外国人を親にもつ子どもは2万4千人に増加しました．小児科診療の視点からは，両親ともに外国人であり日本で出生した子どもも重要です．日本における外国人の人口動態をまとめた人口動態統計特殊報告によると，2007年には13,429人の外国人の出生が報告されています．これを合わせると，父母ともに外国人あるいは父母のどちらかが外国人という子どもは約3万7千人，日本で出生した新生児全体の約3.4％にのぼります．約29人の新生児のうち1人は，外国人の親をもっているということです．

　外来で診療している実感以上に，外国人の子どもが増えていることがわかります．外国人の場合，どこのクリニックに行けばいいのかわからない，いくら医療費がかかるのかわからない，といった理由で，少しくらいの病気ならば，家庭で市販薬や自国から持参した薬でケアしている場合も少なくありません．乳幼児健診にポルトガル語の通訳者を1人導入しただけで，外国人の受診率が急激に高まったという愛知県小牧市の事例もあります．保健医療の現場に外国人の姿が見えないときは，外国人がいないと即断するのではなく，医療へのアクセスが悪いのではないかと疑う必要もありそうです．

　外国人あるいは国際結婚した日本人とその子どもが日本社会の一員として地域で暮らすようになった時代において，出身国の文化やコミュニティを尊重しつつ，どのように質の高い小児保健医療を提供していくのか．まさに，多文化共生社会のあり方が問われています．

2．多文化社会の最前線としての小児科診療

　病院や診療所を外国人の子どもが受診したときに，どうすればいいのでしょうか．

　（母親が外国人で日本語が話せなくても，父親が日本人なら，子どもは日本国籍をもっています．しかし，本稿では，親のひとりが外国人の場合には「外国人の子ども」という表現を使うことにします）．

　小児科の医療現場では，他の診療科と異なり，大きなメリットがあります．診察や看護の場で医師や看護師は，乳幼児や子どもがたとえ一言もしゃべらなくても，その子の状態を把握し的確に診断することができます．ふだんから，言葉だけに頼らずに，子どもの様子や仕草など

1. 外国人の子どもを診察するということ

を通じてコミュニケーションしているからです．言葉の通じない外国人の子どもに対する診療の場合も，日本人の子どもを診ているのと同じように診察すればいいわけです．子どもたちの世界に国境はないのですから．

ただ，外国人の保護者がやってきたときには，出身国，日本での滞在年数，日本語や英語の会話能力などによって，対応の仕方が異なってきます．具体的には，「言語・コミュニケーション」「保険・経済的な問題」「保健医療システムの違い」「異文化理解」という4つの要素に配慮する必要があります．

1）言語・コミュニケーション：きちんとした日本語の大切さ

日本に長期滞在している外国人を対象に，日本の母子保健医療に関するインタビュー調査をしたとき，多くの外国人は，話をよく聞いてくれ，やさしい日本語で説明してくれることを望んでいました．生活のなかでは，電車に乗ったり，コンビニで買い物をしたり，かなりの程度の日本語を使って暮らしています．しかし，少しくらい日本語が話せるからといって，医学用語はむつかしいといいます．高血圧ではなくて，「血圧が高い」という．頭囲といわずに，「頭の大きさ」という．簡単なことで，外国人の親はよく理解してくれるようになります．

主語を省略しないで，きちんとした日本語を使うようにすることも重要です．また，なるべく短い文章で話すように心がけてください．診察室で，お母さんに向かって「歩けますか？」と質問したとき，日本人の母親なら，間違いなく自分の子どもが歩けるようになったかどうか，という質問だと理解してくれます．これは，小児科の診察室という場面設定のなかで，医師と患者の間に暗黙知が作用して，子どもに対する質問だと母親が即座に反応してくれるからです．ところが，外国人の母親の場合には，「私が歩けるかどうかということを，どうしてお医者さんは聞くのだろう」と受け取られることもあります．私自身の失敗談ですが，問診のあと外国人のお母さんの顔を見ながら，「じゃあ，服を脱いでください！」と言ったら，お母さん自身が自分の服を脱ごうとしました．大慌てで「子どもの服をあなたが脱がしてあげてください」と言い直したことがありました．

そういう失敗を経験したいまでは，「お名前はいえますか？」「歩けますか？」といった表現は避けて，「あなたのお子さん（○○ちゃん）は自分の名前がいえますか？」，「あなたのお子さん（○○ちゃん）は歩くことができますか？」と主語と述語が入った，きちんとした文章を話すようにしています．

質問は必ずひとつずつするようにします．一度に，あれもこれも聞くと，相手が混乱します．また，相手の答えが期待したものと異なっているときは，聞き違えている可能性があります（母語でない言語で，わざと質問をはぐらかして答えるというのは，かなり高度なテクニックなので，その可能性は非常に低いです）．そのときには，もう一度聞き方を変えて質問してください．

病院や診療所で作っている案内文や病気の説明文には，漢字にルビを振るようにします．嘔吐（おうと），嚥下（えんげ）障害などの医学用語は，日本人でも読めない人が少なくありません．医学用語にルビを振ると，若いお母さん方からも非常に好評でした．外国人にとって読みやすい案内や説明文は日本人にとっても役立つことがわかりました．

小児科診療では，きちんとした問診を取ることが非常に重要です．基本的な問診事項は，会話で一つずつ聞き出すよりも，あらかじめ作成しておいたチェックリストに記入してもらうほうがお互いの負担が少なくて時間の節約にもなります．いまでは，多くの言語による問診票が，インターネット上で簡単に入手できるようになりました（**表1**）．とくに，「多言語医療問診票」は使いやすいと思います．また，予防接種の問診票としては，予防接種リサーチセンターのホームページが有用です．

表 1　外国語での診療に役立つ冊子・Web サイト

1）**多言語医療問診票**（国際交流ハーティ港南台，かながわ国際交流財団）http://www.k-i-a.or.jp/medical/index.html 　内科，眼科，小児科など 11 の診療科に対応した問診票がダウンロードできる．英語はもとより，スペイン語，ポルトガル語，中国語，ロシア語，フランス語，タイ語，インドネシア語，タガログ語，ベトナム語など 14 言語に対応．
2）**医療機関用外国人ハンドブック**（群馬県医師会）http://www.gunma.med.or.jp/ 　群馬県医師会ホームページの「外国人ハンドブック」から，英語，ポルトガル語，スペイン語，タガログ語の PDF ファイルがダウンロードできる．外来だけでなく，入院，検査，会計，請求書など必要な情報が日本語併記でコンパクトにまとめられている．
3）**多言語生活情報**（自治体国際化協会）http://www.clair.or.jp/tagengo/index.html 　外国人住民の暮らしに関する情報を解説している．「医療」や「出産・育児」では，日本のシステムが簡潔に説明されている．英語，中国語，韓国語，スペイン語，ポルトガル語，タガログ語に対応．
4）**外国語版母子健康手帳**（母子衛生研究会） 　厚生労働省令に基づく母子健康手帳の記録ページを，外国語と日本語の 2 言語で併記．英語，中国語，タガログ語，スペイン語，ポルトガル語，韓国語，タイ語，インドネシア語，ベトナム語．
5）**外国人向け多言語説明資料**（日本医療教育財団：厚生労働省）(http://www.mhlw.go.jp/stf/seisakunitsuite/bunya/0000056789.html) 　院内でよく使われる同意書（手術，麻酔，CT 検査など）や高額医療費制度や出産一時金などについて，英語・中国語・ポルトガル語・スペイン語版がホームページ上からダウンロードできる．問診票だけは日本語と併記されている．

　外国語版母子健康手帳は，小児科では非常に有用なツールです．1992 年に，東京都母子保健サービスセンター（当時）が日本語と外国語を併記する形の外国語版母子健康手帳を日本で初めて開発しました．日本語版の単なる翻訳ではなく，外国語と併記することにより，外国語がわからない保健医療関係者も記入でき，外国人と日本人の夫婦も共通に理解することが可能になりました．現在は，母子衛生研究会が 8 か国語で日本語併記の母子健康手帳を発行しています．多くの自治体でも配布されていますが，母子健康手帳の存在を知らない外国人妊婦に十分に周知されているとはいえません．自治体で配布していない地域では，直接，出版社から購入することも可能です．母子健康手帳をもっていない外国人の母親には，医療関係者が母子健康手帳の取得を勧める必要があります．

　また，外国人の受診者が多い医療機関では，「多言語生活情報」や「日本の母子保健医療・子育てガイド」など，日本の母子保健医療サービスに関する外国語での説明文書を置いておくと重宝します．

　日本語のできない外国人に対して，日本人と同じ水準の医療を提供するためには，ひとりひとりの外国人の病歴，主訴，診断告知，治療方針の説明などに関して十分なコミュニケーションが必要不可欠になります．そのためには，単なるマニュアルやパンフレットだけでは不十分で，保健医療分野に造詣の深い通訳者が必要になります．当然ですが，外国人に対するインフォームド・コンセントは十分な言語理解なしには成立しません．今後，医療現場における通訳者のニーズは急激に増大すると思われます．

　やさしい日本語，正確な問診，母子健康手帳の活用，医療費の情報提供など，外国人の保護者を念頭に，実際の診療場面でのヒントを述べてきました．実は，これらの事項を実践すれば，日本人の保護者にも大変役立つと思います．医師が使う日本語は，日本人にもきちんと理解されているとは限りません．わかりやすい言葉を使うことは当然ですが，他者と十分にコミュニケーションする能力が求められています．

1．外国人の子どもを診察するということ

2）保険・経済的な経済な問題

　基本的には外国人登録を行っていれば，原則として，保健医療に関する種々のサービスは日本人と同様に適用されます．ただ，健康保険への加入資格があるにもかかわらず，実際に加入していない外国人は少なくありません．

　また，オーバーステイといわれる超過滞在者に対する母子保健医療サービスの適応については，2000年に森喜朗内閣総理大臣（当時）が回答した答弁書が公式な政府見解になっています．それによれば，「外国人登録を受けていない外国人が妊娠の届出を行う場合の届出先は，居住地の市町村とすることが適当であり，当該市町村が母子健康手帳を交付することとなる」とされ，超過滞在者も母子健康手帳を受け取ることができます．養育医療に関しては，「医師が入院養育を必要と認めた場合には，在留資格の有無にかかわらず」給付を受けられるとし，育成医療についても「緊急に手術等を行わなければ将来重度の障害を残すような場合には」給付が可能であるという見解を明示しています．

　このように，人道的な見地から，子どもの医療や健康に対する配慮が行われています．ただ，この答弁書の存在を知らない自治体も少なくないので，外国人の子どもの権利を守るためには医療関係者も現状を把握しておく必要があります．

　医療費に関して，明確な情報を提供することが重要です．外国人に対するインタビュー調査で，小児科を受診した母親が語っていました．

　「日本の病院を受診したとき，医者も看護師さんも親切にしてくれて，とてもよかった．でも，最後に会計の前で待っているときが一番緊張した．診察の間ずっと，医療費がどのくらいかかるのかということを誰も話してくれなかったから……」

　私は，「医療費はこれくらいかかるけれど，それでもいいですか」と診察中に医療費のことを率直に話すことにしていました．高価な抗菌薬ではなく，安価な一般薬を選択する患者さんもいました．子どもに対する高額な検査は給料が出てからにしてほしいと申し出た父親もいました．入院を勧めるときも，大体の入院期間と費用を見積もり，その額を事前に伝えていました．このように医療費に関する情報を率直に提供することによって，医療費にまつわるトラブルをかなり回避できたような気がします．

　また，民間の保険に加入している外国人も少なくありません．多くの民間会社の保険では，医療機関において患者が現金で支払い，後日，保険会社が本人に還付するというシステムをとっています．したがって，医療側とすれば，自費診療の患者を診察すると考えればいいわけです．ただ，高価な検査や治療については，保険でカバーできるかどうか確認しておくほうがいいと思います．

3）保健医療システムの違い

　日本で暮らす在住外国人にとって，日本の母子保健医療システムは複雑で理解しにくいようです．とくに，出身国に存在しない保健医療サービスについては，知らないというよりもそのようなサービスが利用できると全く思っていないのがふつうです．日本は世界的に見ても，母子保健サービスの充実した国です．母親学級，妊婦検診，母子健康手帳，先天性代謝異常検査，新生児訪問，乳幼児健診と妊娠，出産，育児の時期に，多くの母子保健サービスが原則として無料で提供されています．諸外国では，これらの母子保健サービスの一部を実施しているにすぎません（表2）．したがって，先進国や途上国を問わず，日本で初めて出産や子育てをする母親にとっては，種々の母子保健医療サービスの存在さえ知らないことも少なくありません．

　たとえば，妊婦検診，出産時の記録，子どもの健診記録や成長が1冊の母子健康手帳としてまとめられているのは，韓国，タイ，インドネシア，ベトナム，ラオス，ユタ州（米国），チュ

表2　日本と諸外国における母子保健医療サービス

項目	日本	先進国	途上国
家族計画	有料	有料	無料
母親学級	ある	国により異なる	実施していない
母子健康手帳	ある	ない	一部の国のみ
先天性代謝異常検査	ある	項目数が少ない	ない
新生児訪問	ある	一部の国のみ	ない
乳幼児健診	集団健診	個別健診	集団健診
予防接種	無料	どちらもある	無料
学校検診	ある	ない	ない

ここでいう先進国と途上国の区別は，厳格なものではない．一応，先進国は北米，西ヨーロッパ，韓国，香港，シンガポールなどを意味し，途上国とはそれ以外の国々を想定している．

ニジア，パレスチナなど非常に限られた国だけです．日本には母子健康手帳というものがあり，子どもの健康や予防接種の記録として有用だという情報を提供する必要があります．

　また，外国人に日本の保健医療システムを説明するときに，日本人用に作られたパンフレットやリーフレットを単に翻訳するだけでは十分ではありません．子どもがけいれん重積を起こしたときに，父親がお金を持って帰宅するのを待っていたフィリピン人のお母さんがいました．救急車を呼ぶには，お金がかかると思い込んでいたのでした．途上国では，救急車は民間病院が運用していることが多く，有料の地域が多いようです．ですから，外国人には，「日本では，救急車は無料です」と伝える必要があります．

　外国人住民の暮らしに関する情報については，自治体国際化協会の「多言語生活情報」が役立ちます．出産・子育てに関する手続きや行政サービスについては，「日本の母子保健医療・子育てガイド」が使いやすいです．医療関係者は，これらの外国人のための冊子などを活用して，日本の乳幼児健診や予防接種のシステムを，聞かれなくても説明してあげるという姿勢が求められています．個人的な経験則では，トラブルが起きてから時間を費やして解決に奔走するよりも，事前にきちんと説明しておいた方がいい，といえます．

3．外国の文化を理解する

　「乳幼児健診で医師がかわいいと思ってタイ人の子どもの頭をつい左手で撫でたら，わが子を侮辱されたとお母さんが感じた」，「かぜをひくからといって夏でも赤ちゃんをグルグル巻きにしている中国人のお母さんにどう保健指導したらいいのかわからない」，といった体験談は少なくありません．

　東南アジアや南アジアの人びととは，日常生活において，左手でものを渡したり，握手したりすることは，一切行っていません．左手は，不浄の手と考えられています．また，タイでは，子どもの頭には精霊が宿っているといわれ，子どもの頭をなでることはタブーです．採血のときに泣かなかった子どもに対して，「えらいね」といって，タイ人の子どもの頭を左手でなでたら，きっと，その母親はすごい剣幕で医師をにらんでいるはずです．

　保育所での調査では，日本人も中国人の母親もほとんどが同じように，子どもの健康に留意していると答えてくれました．ところが，日本人の母親は，活発に動けるようにできるだけ薄着にしているのに対して，中国人の母親は，かぜをひかないようにできるだけ厚着させていると回答したのでした．同じ保育所に通い，同じように子どものためにと思いながら，正反対の

行動になるのです．

　国や地域が異なれば，当然，文化や習慣も異なります．医療者は，民族学者ではないので，それらのすべての文化に精通しておく必要はありません．しかし，自分の行った行為が知らない間に相手を傷つけているかもしれないという感性はもっておきたいものです．異文化との接触の黎明期には，このような種々のコミュニケーションの齟齬が生じるのが当たり前と割り切って考えたほうがいいと思います．

　入浴や手洗いの習慣などの衛生観念が違う，家族の見舞いが多く病床で騒ぐ，ピアスや飾りなどの身体装飾を外さない，など医療側からの苦情は少なくありません．しかし，外国人からみれば，日本もまた固有の文化と習慣を持った国です．日本人と結婚した英国人の妊婦が，妊娠中期の腹帯だけは絶対にしたくないと強く主張し，ついに姑も巻き込んだ家庭争議にまで発展したこともありました．そのときは，初詣に神社にいっても改宗したわけではないように，日本の伝統文化だと思って一日だけ腹帯をしてもらうという妙な妥協策に納得してもらいました．

　こういう混乱の過程を経て，お互いの文化を尊重した相互理解が少しずつ成立していくのだと思います．

　実は，日本人においても，個人の信条や嗜好，宗教的信念によって，病気になったときの行動は一人ひとり異なっています．多くの医療機関では画一的な患者管理が行われ，病院内は規則ずくめといっても過言ではありません．その規則から逸脱した行為を行う個人が日本人であれば個人の問題として考えますが，外国人であれば「外国人の診療は大変である」という偏見につながっている面もあるかもしれません．

　日本人に対しても，一人ひとりの個人の生活スタイルや信条を尊重した医療を実践すれば，外国人の患者との間で生じている異文化摩擦はもっと少なくなるのではないかと期待しています．

Column 1

国際会議で病名が通じなかった

　私は，国際協力機構(JICA)や国連難民高等弁務官事務所(UNHCR)などで仕事をしてきました．その仕事仲間の多くは医療関係以外の人で，外交官，弁護士，ビジネスマン，教育関係者などでした．

　ある国連の会議で，「最近，難民の間でbronchitis(気管支炎)やpneumonia(肺炎)が増加している」と報告したら，みんながキョトンとした顔をしていました．私は，自分の英語の発音が悪いのではないかとあせりました．でも，同席していた保健関係者がrespiratory infection(呼吸器感染症)と言い直すと，国連関係者の皆さんは理解してくれました．

医療関係者が使う英語の診断名は，業界用語にすぎないことを知らされました．

　今では，医療関係者以外の専門家が集まる会議では難しい医療用語は使わず，ラテン語に語源をもつ病名はなるべく別の言葉に置きかえて，話すようにしています．そうすると，少しくらい発音が悪くても，相手が理解してくれるようになりました．

　日本では，英語で学会発表をする訓練は行われていますが，英語で患者さんにやさしく病態を説明するという教育を受けた人は少数にすぎません．とくに医療関係者以外の人と話す場合には，自分の話している英語が難しすぎる(！)場合もあることを知っておく必要があるかもしれません．

（中村安秀）

2章

英語で子どもを診る
（英語を使った小児科診療・総論）

To examine the patient

The aim of this chapter

さまざまな場面を想定した，実用英語集．
よく使う用語ややりとりは「例文」でチェックし，実際の場面で想定される「会話例」で再確認できます．

Part 2　2. 英語で子どもを診る：英語を使った小児科診療・総論

1 あいさつ

　外国で病気になったら，言葉の心配が伴うので誰でも自国で病気になる以上に不安に陥ることでしょう．そんなときに，最初に自分が理解できる言葉であいさつをしてもらったら，それだけでもホッと安心できるでしょう．

　日本では，お医者さんが診察時に自分の名前を名乗るということはあまりないかもしれませんが，たとえばアメリカの診察室では初対面の患者さんに，「Hello, I'm Dr. ○○.」と，自己紹介をすることが多いようです．患者さんの状態がそれほど悪くない場合には，「Nice to meet you.」と握手をして挨拶を交わすということも通常行われています．「初めまして」として習った「How do you do?」というのは，現代ではあまり使われていないようです．

　次に，受診の目的をたずねますが，この場合に気をつけなければならないのは，日本語での「どうされましたか？」という質問を訳すのに，「What is the matter with you ?」と言ってしまいがちですが，これは「どうしたんだ？　何があったの？」というようなニュアンスがあるため，診察室では好ましくありません．

　通常「How can I help you ?」や「What seems to be your problem ?」とたずねますが，「What brought (brings) you here today ?」という，いかにも英語らしい表現もあります．

　再診の場合「Nice to see you again.」というのを日本語で直訳すると，まるで患者さんがまた来たのを喜んでいるような感じを受けますが，英語では患者さんの状態がそれほど悪くない場合には，一般的に使われているようです．

　また，診察が終わったときの挨拶としては「See you again.」や「See you soon.」とは言いませんが，予約などが入っている場合には，「See you next Monday.」とか，「See you next week.」と言います．

　日本語の「おだいじに」という表現に相当するのは，「Take care. I hope you will get well soon.」といった表現ですね．ここでは，「I hope」というのが大切で，「You will get well soon.」と言うと，治ることを100％保証しているようなニュアンスになるので注意しないといけません．

　週末や祝日に近い場合に「Have a nice weekend!」とか「Have a nice holiday!」というと気が利いていますが，クリスマスに関するあいさつは要注意で，いろいろな宗教の信者がいるため，使わない方がよいと言われています．

　初診時には，受付で保険の有無や種類を確認するということも必要です．通常，日本に1年以上滞在する外国人には国民健康保険，また日本の企業に勤めている場合には社会保険に入る場合もあります．そして，海外の健康保険に入っていたり，旅行者の場合には海外旅行保険に入っていたりすることも多くあります．日本の健康保険は，医療機関で通常通り使用できますが，海外の保険会社の場合には，いったん全額を払って後から償還されるということも多いのでその都度確認する必要があります．保険に入っているというのは，「have health insurance」あるいは「be covered by health insurance」というように cover を使ったりもします．

1. あいさつ

例文

(電話で)	
もしもし，○○クリニックです．	Hello, this is ○○ clinic.
いかがなさいましたか？	How can I help you?
(受付で)	
こんにちは．	Hello!
おはようございます．	Good morning.
こんばんは．	Good after noon.
いかがなさいましたか？	How may I help you?
医療保険はお持ちですか？	Do you have health insurance?
(診察室で)	
おはようございます，○○さん．	Good morning, Ms. ○○.
初めまして．	Nice to meet you.
医師の××です．	I am Dr. ××.
今日はどうなさいましたか？	・What brought you here today?
	・What seems to be your problem today?
(再診時)	
こんにちは．	Nice to see you again.
お加減はいかがですか？	How are you feeling today?
(帰り際に)	
次回は来週の木曜日に来てください．	・See you next Thursday.
	・Please come back next Thursday.
良い週末を！	Have a nice weekend!
楽しい休日を！	Have a nice holiday.
気をつけて．	Please take care.
おだいじに．	・I hope you get well soon.
	・I hope all goes well.

関連用語

小児科　pediatric
初診　first visit
健康保険証　health insurance card
保険に入っている　have health insurance
診察券　patient registration card
予約　appointment

初診時の会話例

受付: （電話で）Plulululu…
はい，○○小児科クリニックです．
どうされましたか？
Hello, this is ○○ pediatric clinic.
How can I help you?

患者の母: 私は，アン・スミスと言います．
5歳の娘が体の具合が悪いようなので，受診したいのですが…．
My name is Anne Smith.
My five-year-old daughter seems to be sick, so I'd like to have her seen by a doctor.

受付: お嬢さんのお名前は？
Will you please tell me your daughter's name?

患者の母: メアリーです．
Her name is Mary.

受付: スミスさん，メアリーちゃんは以前にこのクリニックにいらしたことがありますか？
Mrs. Smith, has Mary ever visited our clinic?

患者の母: いいえ，今回が初めてです．
No. This is her first visit to your clinic.

受付: スミスさんは，何か医療保険をお持ちですか？
Mrs. Smith, do you have any health insurance?

患者の母: はい，国民健康保険があります．
Yes, I have National Health Insurance.

受付: メアリーちゃんも，その保険に入っているのですね？
Is Mary covered by the insurance, too?

患者の母: はい，そうです．
Yes, she is.

受付: わかりました．午前10時半でしたら予約がとれます．それまでにお越しください．
Good. We have a 10：30 a.m. appointment available.
Please bring her to our clinic by then.

患者の母: ありがとうございます．では，その時に．
Thank you. See you then.

1. あいさつ

患者の母： （受付で）
10 時半に娘の受診の予約をしたアン・スミスです．
I'm Anne Smith and my daughter has an appointment at 10：30.

受付： スミスさん，こんにちは．保険証を見せていただけますか？
Hello, Mrs. Smith. Will you please show me your health insurance card?

患者の母： はい，これです．
OK, here it is.

受付： ありがとうございます．
診察券をお作りしますので，椅子にかけてしばらくお待ちください．
Thank you very much.
I will make her registration card, so please have a seat and wait for a while.

Column 2

日本で最初の英語による母親学級

1990 年代のはじめ，東京都母子保健サービスセンターが主催して，日本で最初の英語による母親学級を開催しました．会場には，米国，カナダ，ヨーロッパ，香港などの出身の在日外国人の妊婦さんが集まりました．パートナーの日本人男性の姿もありました．

この母親学級の講師は，日本人医師ではなく，日本に住んでいる外国人看護師や助産師にお願いしました．彼女たちは，母国では registered nurse などの資格を持ったプロフェッショナル．日本での医療資格はないけれども，外国人の母子保健医療に関する知識や経験は日本人以上のものがある，と判断したからでした．

「ハイ！ エブリ・ボディ！」という陽気な掛け声からはじまった母親学級．妊婦体操は，いつのまにかエクササイズという名前に変わっていました．ラテン音楽に合わせて，妊婦さんが大きなお腹をかかえてダンスをしました．赤ちゃんの沐浴指導も，笑い声が絶えません．人形の赤ちゃんに，みんなで水しぶきをかけながらシャワーをしているようでした．

こんなにおおらかで楽しい母親学級は，私にとってもはじめての経験でした．外国人コミュニティのことを熟知しているのは外国人であり，日本にも多くの外国人専門職が暮らしていることを教えられました．外国人の保健医療サービスの充実には，当事者である外国人が主体的に参加できるような場を提供することが重要なのだと思います．

（中村安秀）

Part 2　2．英語で子どもを診る：英語を使った小児科診療・総論

2　症状を聞く

　症状を聞くというのは，診察の第一歩であることは言うまでもありませんね．
　診察室で最初に聞かれる質問といえば，「どうされましたか？」という言葉が浮かんできます．
　この質問を英語で聞く場合に，「What is the matter with you ?」や，「What is wrong with you ?」という聞き方は，直接過ぎて好まれないようです．またこのように聞くと，「それを調べるために来たんですよ」と返事をする患者さんもいるかもしれません．
　そのかわりに，医療の現場では「What seems to be your problem ?」「どのようなことでお困りですか？」や，「What brought you here ?」のように，症状や問題を主語にするという英語らしい表現がよく使われます．
　また，症状を聞くときには，「どのような症状がありますか？」「症状について詳しく述べてください」のように聞きます．
　多くみられる症状の一つに発熱がありますが，熱に関しては「熱はありますか？」「何度くらいありますか？」「熱は上がったり下がったりしますか？」，あるいは「寒気がありますか」などという質問がされます．
　また，熱の単位は多くの国でセ氏（Celsius または Centigrade）を使いますが，例えば米国などではカ氏（Fahrenheit）を使いますので，換算ができるようにしておくと便利でしょう．〔℃ =（°F − 32）× 5/9〕．
　痛みも大事な症状の一つで，「痛みはありますか？」「どのような痛みですか？」と聞きますが，日本人同士でも痛みを相手に伝えるのは難しいですね．英語でもいろいろな答え方がありますが，そのニュアンスを理解するのはかなり難しいです．また痛みの強さについても人それぞれ，感じ方や表現が違うかもしれません．
　英語では痛みの程度を，「mild（弱い）」「moderate（中程度）」「severe（強い）」と表現しますが，下図のような表情の違う顔の絵を使って，Which face describes your pain well?（どの顔があなたの痛みをよく表していますか？）と聞いてみるとわかりやすいかも知れません．
　一方，診察時には，熱，痛みなどのほかに，便や尿についての症状を聞かなければならないことが多くあります．「便通はどうですか？」「下痢・便秘をしていますか？」「便に血が混じっていますか？」「尿が出にくいですか？」「1日に何回くらい排尿しますか？」などといった質問がされるでしょう．

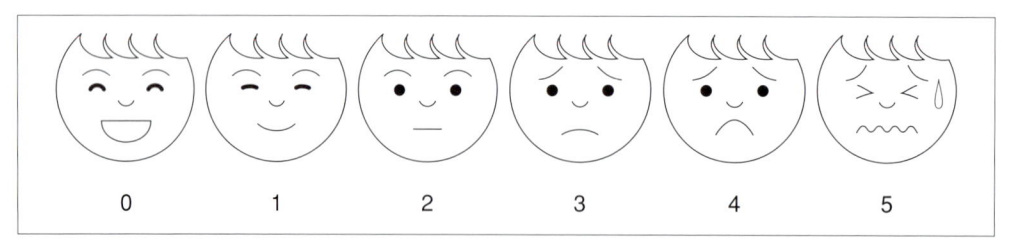

図　ペインチャート

2. 症状を聞く

例文

どうされましたか？	What seems to be your problem?
	What brought you here today?
	What brings you here today?
熱はありますか？	Do you have a fever?
	Do you have a temperature?
熱は何度ありますか？	What is your temperature?
寒気がしますか？	Do you feel chilly?
痛みはありますか？	Do you have pain?
どこが痛みますか？	Where does it hurt?
それはどのような痛みですか？	What kind of pain is it?
痛み止めは効きましたか？	Did a painkiller have any effect?
便通はいかがですか？	What about your bowel movement?
便通は規則的にありますか？	Are your bowel movements regular?
便に血が混じることはありませんか？	Have you ever had blood in your stools?
排便は1日に何回ありますか？	How many bowel movement do you have a day?
便秘をしていますか？	Are you constipated?
下痢をしていますか？	Do you have diarrhea?
排尿時に痛みますか？	Does it hurt when you urinate?
尿が出にくいですか？	Is it difficult to urinate?
尿の色はどうですか？	What is the color of your urine?
症状はいつから始まりましたか？	When did your symptom start?
どのような時に症状は悪く/良くなりますか？	What makes your symptoms worse/better?
症状について，もう少し詳しく述べてください．	Will you please describe your symptoms in more detail?

✓ check Memo　「尿の色」

「尿の色」はだいたい以下で聞き取ることができるでしょう．

- ☐ 澄んでいる　clear
- ☐ 濁っている　cloudy
- ☐ ピンク色　pink
- ☐ 赤褐色　reddish brown
- ☐ 黄褐色　yellowish brown
- ☐ 茶褐色　liver color, dark reddish brown

関連用語

症状　symptom
熱　fever, temperature, body temperature
吐き気　nausea
吐き気がする　nauseous
吐く　vomit
食欲　appetite
寒気，悪寒　chill
痛み　pain
ズキズキする痛み　throbbing pain
我慢できない痛み　unbearable pain
ヒリヒリする痛み　soreness
激痛　severe pain
鈍痛　dull pain
チクチクする(刺すような)痛み　stabbing pain
キリキリする(鋭い)痛み　sharp pain
急性の痛み　acute pain
間欠的な痛み　intermittent pain
慢性的な痛み　chronic pain
ズキンズキンする(脈打つような)痛み　pulsating pain
頭痛　headache
歯痛　toothache
腹痛　stomachache
喉の痛み　sore throat
片頭痛　migraine
生理痛　menstrual pain
痛みの程度(弱，中，強)　mild, moderate, severe
便　stool
便通，排便　bowel movement
便秘　constipation
下痢　diarrhea
血便　bloody stool, hematochezia
尿　urine
血尿　blood in the urine, hematuria
頻尿　frequent urination
排尿する　urinate
尿失禁　urinary incontinence
尿閉　urinary retention, urodialysis
(症状)が続く　persist
悪化する　get worse, deteriorate
(薬が)効く　work

2. 症状を聞く

初診時の会話例

医師: 今日はどうされましたか？
What seems to be your problem today?

患者: 熱があって，おなかも痛いです．
I have a fever and pain in my stomach.

医師: おなかの痛みについて教えてください．
Will you please describe to me about your abdominal pain?
どのような痛みですか？
What kind of pain is it?

患者: チクチクした(刺すような)痛みがずっとくり返している感じです．
It's like a stabbing pain/and it comes and goes.

医師: いつごろから，熱やお腹の痛みがありますか？
When did your fever and pain start?

患者: 一昨日（おととい）からです．
They started the day before yesterday.

医師: 熱を測りましたか？
Did you take your temperature?

患者: はい，今朝は99.5度でした．
Yes, I did. It was 99.5 degrees this morning.

医師: ああ，あなたの国ではカ氏を使われるのですね．
セ氏では大体37.5度になりますね．
Oh, in your country you use Fahrenheit, right?
It's almost 37.5 degrees Celsius.

医師: 下痢または便秘をしていますか？
Do you have diarrhea or constipation?

患者: いつもよりも柔らかいです．
でも水みたいというほどではありません．
My stool is softer than usual
But I wouldn't say it's watery.

医師: 何度くらい排便がありましたか？
How often did your bowel move?

17

患者: 昨日は，4回だったと思います．
I think four times yesterday.

医師: 便に血は混ざっていませんか？
Did you notice blood in your stools?

患者: いいえ，混ざっていません．
No, I didn't. I don't think I had blood in my stools.

医師: 吐き気はどうですか？ あるいは吐きましたか？
Do you have nausea or have you vomited?

患者: 吐き気はありません．
No, I don't have nausea.

医師: 食欲はいかがですか？
How about your appetite?

患者: いつもほどはありません．あまり，お腹も空きません．
I don't have much of an appetite. I don't get hungry as much as usual.

医師: あなたの症状は，悪化していますかそれとも良くなってきていますか？
Do you think your symptoms are getting worse or better?

患者: 残念ながら，悪くなっています．
Unfortunately, they are getting worse.

医師: ご家族で，同じような症状がある人はいますか？
Does anyone in your family have the same symptoms?

患者: いいえ，誰もこのような症状がある人はいません．
No, None of my family has these symptoms.

Part 2　2．英語で子どもを診る：英語を使った小児科診療・総論

3　既往歴を聞く

　既往歴や，現在かかっている病気は，治療方針を決めたり，薬を処方したりする時にとても大切な情報になります．

　また，その病気がいつごろかかったものなのか，今も治療を続けているのか，手術をしたのか，薬で治したのかなど，いろいろと重要な質問がありますし，患者さん本人だけではなく，その家族の既往歴も重要な情報となります．

　さらには，病気だけでなく，薬のアレルギーや副作用が強く出た薬についてなどの質問も既往歴に含まれると言えます．また，これらの質問は問診票の中で聞かれることも多くあります．

　既往歴を聞く場合には，ほとんどが過去のことになるので，英語では「Have you ever…」という現在完了形がよく使われます．また，家族についての質問で，「家族の中にどなたか…」と聞く時には，「Does anyone in your family…」とか，「Has anyone in your family…」と聞くと良いでしょう．この場合の「家族」には，血縁者という意味と，同居の家族という意味があります．とくに遺伝的な病気について問うような，近親の血縁者について問う場合には，close relative という言い方をするとわかりやすいでしょう．ただし，近親の血縁といっても人によって解釈に違いがあるので，具体的に言う方がわかりやすいかも知れません．ちなみに日本では第一親等というと，両親と子どもを指しますが，英語の「first-degree relative（FDR）」は，血がつながった両親，子どもと兄弟姉妹も含み，また「second-degree relatives」には，祖父母，孫，おじ・おば，甥・姪，異父母の兄弟姉妹までを含むようです．これとよく似た「immediate relative」は，血縁に関わらず，両親，子ども，兄弟姉妹，祖父母をはじめ，法的な家族，いわゆる in laws も含むので注意が必要です．

　症状についての質問は数多くあるので，例文を参考に応用してみましょう．

親戚の呼び方

父方のみ記載しましたが，母方も呼び方は同じです．

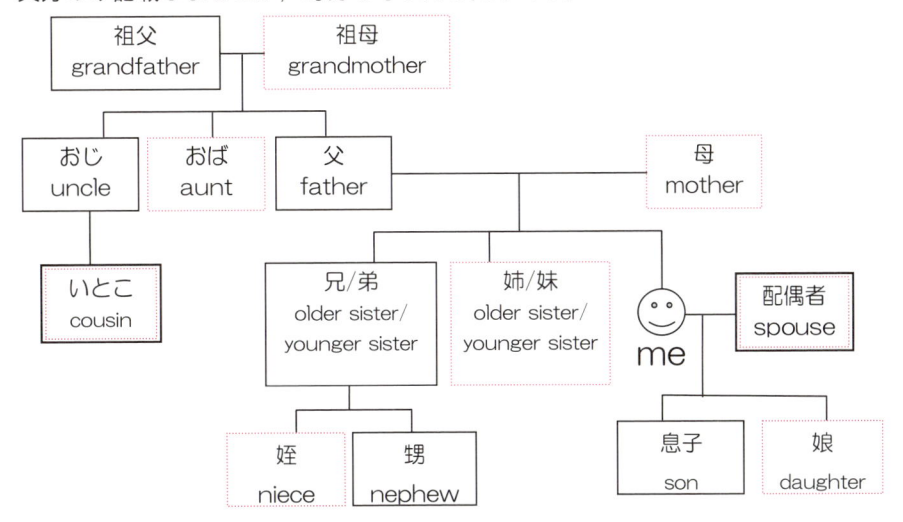

```
                祖父 grandfather ─── 祖母 grandmother
                        │
    ┌───────────┬───────┴─────┐
  おじ uncle   おば aunt      父 father ─── 母 mother
    │                              │
  いとこ cousin            ┌───────┴──────┐
                    兄/弟              姉/妹           me ─── 配偶者 spouse
                    older sister/       older sister/         │
                    younger sister      younger sister        │
                           │                          ┌───────┴──────┐
                    ┌──────┴──────┐                 息子 son    娘 daughter
                   姪 niece      甥 nephew
```

例文

お子さんは，今までにどんな予防接種を受けましたか？	What vaccinations has your child ever gotten?
妊娠中，何か問題はありませんでしたか？	Did you have any problem during pregnancy?
出産時に，何か問題はありませんでしたか？	Did you have any problem during childbirth?
生後，お子さんの成長，発達は順調ですか？	After birth, is your child growing and developing normally?
お子さんは，これまでに何か大きな病気にかかったことがありますか？	Has your child ever had a serious disease?
その病気は，完治していますか？	Has the disease been cured completely?
まだ治療中ですか？	Is your child still being treated for the disease?
薬を飲んで発疹が出たり気分が悪くなったりしたことがありますか？	Has your child ever had a rash or been sick after taking medication?
今までに食物でアレルギーが出たことはありますか？	Has your child ever had an allergic reaction to any foods?
現在，食物アレルギーのために除去している食物はありますか？	Are there any foods you are eliminating from your child diet for food allergy now?
過去に，手術を受けたことがありますか？	Has your child ever had an operation?
今，定期的に何か薬を飲んでいますか？	Is your child taking any medication regularly now?
家族の中に，大きな病気にかかった人がいますか？	Has anyone in your family had a serious illness?
輸血をしたことがありますか？	Has your child ever had a blood transfusion?
麻酔を受けたことがありますか？	Has your child ever had anesthesia?
以前にもこのような症状が見られたことがありましたか？	Has your child ever had this kind of symptom before?
今回のご病気で，他の医療機関にかかられましたか？	Have you taken your child to other hospitals or clinics for this disease?

関連用語

予防接種　vaccination, immunization
妊娠　pregnancy
出産　childbirth
食物アレルギー　food allergy
除去する　eliminate, avoid
高血圧　hypertension, high blood pressure
発疹　rash
糖尿病　diabetes, mellitos
治療する　treat
薬，薬物　medication

インシュリン　insulin
食事療法（治療法の１つとして言う場合）　dietary measure
食事療法（低塩食，低たんぱく食など特定の食事を言う場合）　special diet
ガン　cancer
輸血　blood transfusion
肝機能　liver function
異常　abnormality
麻酔　anesthesia
症状　symptom

3．既往歴を聞く

初診時の会話例

医師: これまでの病歴についてお尋ねします．
I'd like to ask you about your child's medical history.

医師: 今までに，大きな病気をしたことがありますか？
Has your child ever had any serious disease?

患者の母: 大きな病気と言いますと…？
What do you mean by serious disease?

医師: 入院や手術をするような病気と考えていただければよいでしょう．
I mean diseases for which he/she needed to be hospitalized or needed to have an operation.

患者の母: 2年前に肺炎で入院したことがあります．
He/She was hospitalized for pneumonia two years ago.

医師: 今までにお薬を飲んで，気分がわるくなったり発疹が出たりしたことはありますか？
Has he/she ever felt sick or gotten a rash after taking any medication?

患者の母: いいえ，ないと思います．
No. I don't think so.

医師: 何かアレルギーがあると言われたことはありますか？
Has he/she ever been told that he/she has any kind of allergy?

患者の母: 食べ物ではアレルギーはありませんが，毎年春先になると花粉アレルギーが起こります．
He/She is not allergic to any foods, but he/she has a pollen allergy in early spring every year.

医師: これまでに，どのような予防接種を受けられましたか？
What vaccination has he/she ever gotten?

患者の母: 3種混合ワクチンとポリオの生ワクチンを受けました．
He/She has been inoculated with DPT and Polio vaccine.

医師: それらの予防接種を受けた時に，何か問題はありませんでしたか？
Did he/she have any problem when he/she got the vaccination?

患者の母: いいえ，ありませんでした．
No, he/she didn't have.

Part 2　2. 英語で子どもを診る：英語を使った小児科診療・総論

4　診察する

　次は，いよいよ診察に入ります．
　診察を始めるとき，まずお医者さんは「では診てみましょう」とか，「では診させてください」と言います．これは，「I will examine you.」という少し硬い言い方でもよいのですが，「Let me take a look.」や，「Let me take a look at you.」のような決まり文句があります．
　また，診察時には，服を脱いだり，横になったり，息を吸ったり吐いたりと，患者さんにもいろいろと指示が出されます．簡単なことですが，いざ外国語にするとなると，どのように言うのだろうと考えてしまう表現が多いですね．使われる英単語自体はそれほど難しいものは必要ありません．忘れてはいけないのは，指示を出すときに，「please」を付けたり，「I'd like you to………．」と丁寧に話すことですね．
　外国人の患者さんの場合，文化や宗教についての配慮も大切です．たとえばイスラム教の文化では，女性の患者さんを男性のお医者さんが診察するということは本当にまれなことで，場合によっては拒否する患者さんもいらっしゃいます．とくに，肌を見せなければならないような診察は，女性のお医者さんを強く希望されることがあります．
　また，婦人科の検診の際に，日本ではお医者さんと患者さんの間にカーテンのような仕切りを置いて，直接顔が見えないようにしますが，国によってはお医者さんの顔が見えないと不安に思われる患者さんもいらっしゃるようです．
　日本ではお医者さんが聴診器を使って胸の診察をしたり背中の音を聴いたりするときに，患者さんが自分の椅子を回して，指示通りに動きますが，外国では患者さんは診察台や椅子に座ったままで，お医者さんが移動して背中を診たりするのが普通のところもあります．
　外国人の患者さん一人ひとりの文化を理解したり希望を聞き入れたりすることは大変なことですが，少しでも安心して診察が受けられるような配慮をすれば，その気持ちは患者さんにも伝わるでしょう．

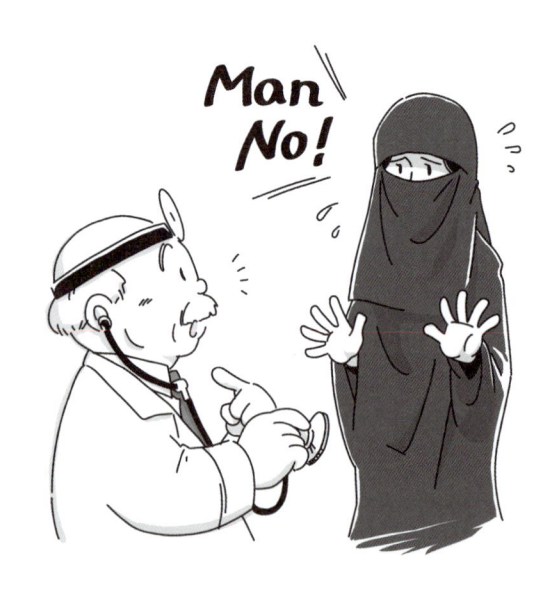

4．診察する

例文

診察をします．	Let me take a look at you.
上半身を脱いでください．	Please take off your clothes from the waist up.
下半身を脱いでください．	Please take off your clothes from the waist down.
右袖をまくってください．	Please roll up your right sleeve.
喉を診ます．	Let me take a look at your throat.
口を大きく開けて，"ア〜"と言ってください．	Please open your mouth wide and say "ahh".
舌を出してください．	Stick out your tongue please.
息を大きく吸って，吐いてください．	Take a deep breath, now let it out.
息を吸って止めてください．	Breathe in and hold please.
診察台の上に仰向けに寝てください．	Please lie down on your back on the examination table.
診察台の上にうつ伏せになってください．	Please lie face down on the examination table.
膝を曲げて，お腹を楽にしてください．	Bend your knees and relax your abdomen, please.
背中を診ますので反対側を向いてください．	Turn around, please. I'd like to check your back.
ここを押すと痛いですか？	Does it hurt when I press here?
左目をつむってください．（眼科）	Please close your left eye.
このラインの上をまっすぐに歩いてください．	Please walk straight along this line.
腱反射を診ます．	I will check your tendon reflexes.
首を触って，甲状腺を診ます．	I'm going touch your neck to examine your thyroid.
服を着てください．	Please get dressed.

関連用語

診察　examination
息を吸う　breathe in, inhale
息を吐く　breathe out, exhale
息を止める　hold one's breath
仰向けに寝る　lie on one's back, lie face up
仰向けに寝かせる　lay someone on one's back
うつ伏せに寝る　lie on one's stomach, lie face down
うつ伏せに寝かせる　lay someone on one's stomach
左(右)向きに寝る　lie on one's left(right) side
左(右)向きに寝かせる　lay someone on one's left(right) side
腱反射　tendon reflex
聴診器　stethoscope
診察台　examination table

初診時の会話例

医師: では診察をします.
Let me take a look.
上半身の服を脱いでください.
Please take off your clothes from the waist up.

患者: はい, 先生.
OK, doctor.

医師: 聴診器で, 胸の音を聴きます.
I will listen to your chest with my stethoscope.
大きく息を吸って, …吐いて…, もう一度吸って….
Take a deep breath, and breathe out, breathe in again….
次に, 背中を診ますので, 反対を向いてください.
Turn around, please. I'd like to check your back.
はい, 大きく息を吸って…, 吐いて…, 吸って…, そこで息を止めてください.
OK, please take a deep breath…, breathe out…, breathe in again and hold your breath.
はい, いいですよ. 楽にして.
OK, you can breathe out/exhale now and please relax.
もう一度こちらを向いてください.
Please turn around and look at me.
喉を診ますので, 大きく口を開けて「アー」と言ってください.
Please open your mouth wide and say "ahh".
今度は, 首を触って甲状腺が腫れていないかを診ます.
Next, I will palpate your neck to see if your thyroid is swollen.
異常はないようですね.
I don't feel any abnormality.
次に, お腹を診ます. 診察台に仰向けに寝てください.
Next, I'd like to examine your abdominal area.
Please lie face up on the examination table.

患者: 頭はどちらですか？
At which end should my head go?

医師: 頭はこちらの端になるように寝てください.
Please lie down with your head at this end.
お荷物はかごの中に入れてくださいね.
Use this basket for your things, please.
そしてベルトを緩めてください.
Please loosen your belt.
はい, 膝を曲げて, お腹を楽にして.
OK, bend your knees and relax your abdomen, please.

4．診察する

ここを押さえると痛みますか？　あるいは，吐き気がしたりしますか？
Does it hurt when I press here? Or do you feel nauseous?

患者: いいえ，大丈夫です．
No. I'm OK.

医師: ここはどうですか？
How about this area?

患者: 少し痛みます．
It hurts a little.

医師: 私がお腹を押したときに痛みますか？　それとも，手を離すときに痛みますか？
Do you feel pain when I press your abdomen or when I remove my hand?

患者: 離すときに痛むようです．
When you remove your hand, I think.

医師: はい，結構です．
OK, I'm done.
服を着てください．
Please get dressed.

Column 3

背中の引っかき傷—虐待と間違えないで—

　ベトナムの家庭では，カゼをひいたり，熱があったりすると，硬貨（コイン）やヘラを使って，背中をこすります．脊柱から外に向かって，思いっきりガリガリと引っかくのです．背中には，内出血を起こした赤い傷が何本も残ります．そして，薬効があるといわれるハッカ入りの油を塗りこんで，治療は終了．カゼをひいたときには，とても効果があるといわれています．

　小さな子どもの背中に何本もの引っかき傷があると，はじめてみた人はびっくりします．アメリカ合衆国では，保育所でベトナム人の子どもの背中の傷をみて，児童虐待と間違えたといわれています．

　このカオヨー，あるいはカオゾーという民間療法．ベトナム人と結婚した日本人の間では好評のようです．ベトナム人の子どもの背中に引っかき傷を見つけたときは，伝統療法なのかもしれません．

（中村安秀）

Part 2　2. 英語で子どもを診る：英語を使った小児科診療・総論

5　検査をしましょう

　検査は，現代の医療には不可欠のものとなっています．
　検査についての説明には，検査そのものを説明するものと，患者さんに指示を出すための説明があります．たとえば前者には，「検査をする意義」「検査の方法やかかる時間」「検査に伴う危険性」などがありますが，造影剤を使う検査などでは，同意書などに署名を求めることがあるので，説明も膨大なものになるでしょう．
　一方後者には，採血の際の袖をまくる動作の指示から，「呼吸の仕方」「身体の位置」の指示などがあります．検査を正確かつスムーズに行なうためには，外国語であっても的確に指示を出すことが大切ですが，日本語では簡単な表現なのに，外国語の場合にはなかなか出てこないということは多々ありますね．たとえば，バリウムを使って胃のエックス線を撮る検査などでは，患者さんは検査技師の指示にしたがって動かないといけない上にバリウムはどんどん流れて行ってしまうので，迅速にさらにわかりやすく患者さんに指示を出す必要があります．日ごろから使い慣れておかないととっさに言葉が出てこないということになりますね．
　検査日の絶食や持ち物などの指示なども正しく伝えておかないと，正しい検査結果が得られず，あるいは当日に検査が受けられずに二度手間になるなどということもあるので，気をつけなければなりません．
　また，検査には高額の費用がかかるものもありますので，後でトラブルにならないように，事前にきちんと説明しておくことも大切です．
　次に，検査時に使われる代表的な表現を紹介します．

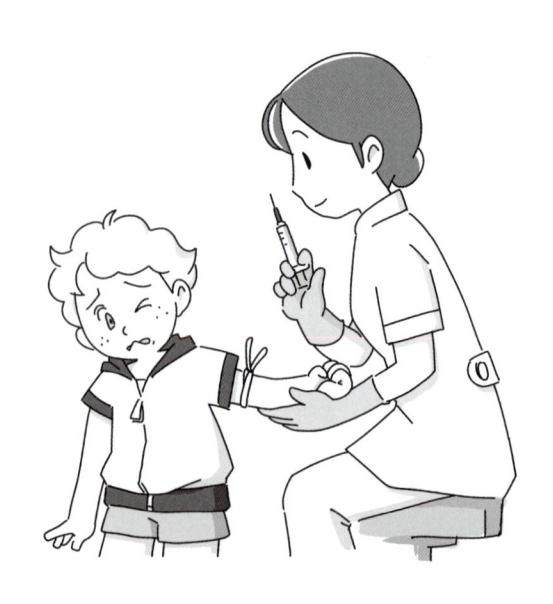

5．検査をしましょう

例文

採血をします．	I'm going to take a blood sample.
右腕の袖をまくって，腕を前に出してください．	Please roll up your right sleeve and put your arm out.
血圧を測ります．	I'm taking your blood pressure.
すこしチクッとしますよ．	This may hurt a little.
親指を中に入れて，拳をつくってください．	Please make a fist with your thumb inside.
尿検査をします．	I'll give you a urine test.
最初の尿を捨てて，中間の尿を採ってください．	Please urinate into the toilet first and then take a sample of midstream.
エックス線を撮りますので，呼ばれるまでエックス線室の前で待っていてください．	We are going to take a chest X-rays, so please wait in front of the X-ray room.
聴力検査をします．	I'm going to check your hearing.
音が聞こえたら，このボタンを押してください．	Please press this button when you hear a sound.
上部消化管のバリウム検査をします．前の夜は，9時までに夕食を済ませておいてください．	You are going to have an Upper GI series. Please don't eat anything after 9:00 pm on the night before.
この輪のどの部分が開いているかを指で示してください．	Please show me which part of this circle is open with your finger.
アレルゲンを調べるために，プリックテストをします．	I'll give you a skin prick test to identify the allergen.
腎臓の超音波検査をします．	I'm going to do an ultrasound of your kidneys.
お腹にジェルを塗りますので，少し冷たいかもしれません．	I'll put gel on your stomach, so it may feel a little cold.

関連用語

- 血圧　blood pressure
- 血液検査　blood test
- 尿検査　urine test
- エックス線撮影　X-ray
- 上部消化管造影検査　Upper GI (Gastro-Intestinal) series
- 検査着　examination gown
- バリウム　barium
- 心電図　ECG, electrocardiogram
- 電極　electrode
- 超音波検査　ultrasonography, echography, ultrasound
- CT　computer tomogram, CT scan
- 内視鏡検査　endoscopic exam, endoscopy
- 脳波　EEG, electroencephalogram
- 喀痰検査　sputum examination
- 精密検査　thorough examination
- 生検　biopsy
- 便潜血検査　occult blood test
- 末梢血酸素飽和度　Saturation of Peripheral Oxygen (SpO2), Sat level
- 視力検査　vision examination, eye test
- 聴力検査　audibility test, hearing test

初診時の会話例

技師

(心電図)

これから心電図をとりますので，上半身の服と靴を脱いで診察台に上がって下さい．頭はこちらの端です．靴下も脱いで下さい．
Before I take the electrocardiogram, please take off your shoes. Please also take off your clothes from the waist up and your stockings, then lie on your back on the examination table with your head at this end.

身体の力を抜いて楽な姿勢をとって下さい．検査中は動いたり，話したりしないで下さい．
Please lie in a relaxed and comfortable position, and please don't move or speak during the test.

では，両方の手足と胸に電極を着けます．少し冷たいですよ．
I'll place electrodes onto the skin on both arms, both legs, and your chest. They may feel a little cold.

検査は5分程かかります．検査が終わったら，電極を取りはずします．
The whole procedure will take about five minutes. After the test, the electrodes will be removed.

終わりました．服を着て下さい．
We're finished. You can get dressed.

技師

(超音波検査)

超音波検査の前に，お腹にゼリーを塗ります．ちょっと冷たいですよ．
Before the ultrasound, I will put some gel on your stomach. It may feel a little cold.

看護師

(血液検査)

今から，血液検査のために少し血液を取ります．
I will draw blood for a blood test.

片方の袖をまくって腕を台の上に乗せてください．
Roll up one of your sleeves and put your arm on this table.

親指を中に入れて握りこぶしを作って，じっとしてください．はい，力を抜いて．
Make a fist with your thumb inside of it, and don't move. OK, relax your arm.

終わりました．絆創膏を貼りますので，もまないでしっかり上から押さえておいてください．
I've finished. I will put a bandage. Don't rub the area but press firmly.

技師

(上部消化管造影)

上半身の衣服をすべて脱いで，この検査着を着てください．
Please take off your clothes from your waist up and wear this gown.

次に，この顆粒をこの水で飲んでください．これは，胃の内部でガスを発生させて胃を膨らませるためのものです．飲むとゲップをしたくなりますが，がまんしてください．

5．検査をしましょう

Next, please take these granules with this water. They will generate gas in your stomach and inflate it. You may feel as if you need to burp, but please don't.

次に，機械のふみ台の上に上がって下さい．検査中台を動かしますので，両手で左右の手すりをしっかりと握ってください．

Then, please step onto the platform of this X-ray machine. I will rotate the machine, so please hold on to the handrails with both hands.

では，始めます．

Now, let's start.

台の横のカップの中にあるバリウムを少し含んで，はい，次にゆっくりと飲みこんでください．

Take the cup next to the machine and keep a small amount of barium in your mouth, then swallow it.

そして，ゆっくりと左から回ってください．

Please turn from left to right slowly.

はい，そこで止まって大きく息を吸って，止めて動かないで．
はい，結構です．普通に息をしてください．

OK, stop there and take a deep breathe. Hold it and please don't move.
OK. Please breathe normally.

次に，バリウムを全部飲んでください．

Please drink the rest of barium now.

今度は，あなたの右側が前に来るようにもう少し左を向いて．

And please face a little to the left so that your right side comes forward.

はい，そこで止まって大きく息を吸って，息を止めて．はい，結構です．

OK, please stop there and take a deep breathe, hold it. OK.

次に，台を水平の位置まで動かします．落ちないように気をつけて．

Next, I will rotate the table down to the horizontal position.
Be careful not to fall off the table.

そして，今度は2～3回，台の上で回ってください．

Now roll over a couple of times on the table.

はい，そこで止まって．息を止めて．はい，結構です．

OK, stop there, hold your breath. OK.

では，台をもとの位置に戻します．

Now, I will swing the table back to the original position.

これで検査は終了です．

Now, we are done.

今日のバリウムが排泄されるように，看護師が下剤をお渡ししますので，すぐに飲んでおいてください．

The nurse will give you laxatives to help you pass the barium.
So, take them soon.

Part 2　2．英語で子どもを診る：英語を使った小児科診療・総論

6　診断を伝える

　診断を伝えるのは，インフォームド・コンセントの重要な部分です．
　診察をしてすぐに診断がつくような病気もあれば，検査をして出た結果から診断して，後日患者さんに伝えるものもあります．また，治療が必要な場合には治療方法を，そして手術や入院が必要な場合には手術の方法や入院にかかる日数，予後などについても説明しなければいけません．
　「あなたは○○病にかかっています」というのは，「You have ○○病.」といういい方が一般的で，たとえば，「肺炎にかかっています」というのは，「You have pneumonia.」と言います．
　検査結果からはっきりとは断定できないけれども，ある病気が疑われるという場合には，「I suspect you have……」という表現が使われます．
　また，重い病気で患者さんの気持ちを察しながら伝えるときには，「I'm afraid you have…」のような表現を使います．
　検査結果には，いろいろな数値が出てきますが，数値を表す単語には「count」や「level」が使われます．一般に「count」は，血液中の血球の数を表すときに，「level」はコレステロールや血糖の値を表すときに使います．たとえば，「血糖値」は「blood-sugar level」，「コレステロール値」は「cholesterol level」がよく使われていますが，「blood-sugar count」，「cholesterol count」のように「count」を使って表現することもまれにあるようです．
　血圧の数値を伝えるとき，日本語では「血圧の上は130で下が70です．」のように言いますが，英語では，「130 over 70」と，「over」を使って表します．また，その数値は「blood pressure reading」と言います．血圧の単位の「mmHg」は，「millimeters of mercury」と読みますが，通常は数字だけを伝えます．

Column 4

日本語の数字は難しい―"なな"なの？"しち"なの？―

　外国人のお母さんのなかには，流暢に日本語を話す方も少なくありません．ただ，日本語の数字は，外国人には難しいようです．
　「次の診察は，はつか(二十日)にしましょう」
　「お子さんの体重は，じゅうなな(十七)キログラムでした」
　私の言葉に，お母さんから，次のように聞き返されたことがあります．
　　20日をなぜ「はつか」というのですか？
　　「じゅうなな」も「じゅうしち」も同じですか？
　日本語が話せる外国人にも，数字だけはメモ用紙に書き込んで渡すようにしています．ちょっとした手間をかけることで，誤解を生まないで済むなら，それがいちばん．ただ，私が大慌てで「7」と書いたら，「これは何の数字ですか？」と聞いたお母さんがいたので，数字はていねいに書く必要がありそうです．

（中村安秀）

6. 診断を伝える

例文

先日の検査の結果が出ました.	We have the results of the latest test.
先日の検査結果によると……	According to the result
空腹時の血糖値が 140 mg/dL で, 正常値よりも少し高いです.	Your fasting blood-sugar level is 140 mg/dL. It's a little higher than normal.
血圧は, 135/65 mmHg です.	Your blood pressure is 135 over 65.
喉の奥が少し赤いですね.	The back of your throat is a little reddish.
右の首のリンパ腺が腫れています.	The lymph gland on the right side of your neck is swollen.
胸の音はきれいです.	Your chest sounds clear.
胆石の疑いがあります.	I suspect you have gallstones.
入院して, 詳しい検査をしていただきます.	You need to be hospitalized and have a detailed examination.
手術の必要があります.	You need to have surgery.
心臓には異常は認められません.	I don't see any abnormality in your heart.
残念ですが, 検査した細胞5個のうち3個に悪性という結果が出ました.	I'm afraid the result shows that three of the five examined cells are malignant.
コレステロール値が高いです.	Your cholesterol level is high.
薬が効いているとは思えません.	The medications do not seem to be working.
足を骨折しています.	You have a fractured leg.
靱帯が切れています.	Your ligament is torn.
検査で肝機能に異常が認められました.	The examination detected abnormalities in your liver function.
○○先生に紹介状を書きます.	・I will refer you to Dr. ○○. ・I will write a referral form to Dr. ○○ for you.

関連用語

検査結果	result of examination	肺炎	pneumonia
コレステロール値	cholesterol level	高血圧	high blood pressure, hypertension
中性脂肪値	neutral fat level	高コレステロール血症	hyperlipemia, hyperlipidemia
空腹時血糖値	fasting blood-sugar level, fasting blood glucose level	糖尿病	diabetes mellitus
ヘモグロビン A_{1c}	hemoglobin A_{1c}	貧血	anemia
赤血球数	red blood cell count, RBC count	虫垂炎	appendicitis
白血球数	white blood cell count, WBC count	肝炎	hepatitis
腫れている	swollen	腎臓病	kidney disease
肥大している	enlarged	骨折	bone fracture
疑いがある	to be suspected	ねんざ	distortion, sprain
良性	benign	脱臼	dislocation
悪性	malignant	紹介状	referral form

初診時の会話例

医師: 先ほどのエックス線検査の写真ができました．
We have the latest X-rays.

患者の母: 先生，メアリーはどこか悪いのでしょうか？
Doctor, what is wrong with Mary?

医師: （エックス線写真を見せて）肺が白くなっているのが見えますね．
You see the whitish area in her lungs, don't you?

患者の母: ああ，私にもわかります．
Oh, yes. I can see it.

医師: メアリーちゃんは，肺炎を起こしていますね．
She has pneumonia.

患者の母: 肺炎ですか!?
Pneumonia!?

医師: そうです．今，マイコプラズマ肺炎が流行っています．
Yes, Mycoplasma Pneumonia is going around now.

患者の母: マイコ？
Myco…?

医師: マイコプラズマ．マイコプラズマは，細菌の一種と考えてくだされればいいのですが，大きさは細菌とウィルスの間くらいです．細菌が持っている細胞壁というものを持たないのが特徴の病原体です．
Yes, Mycoplasma. Mycoplasma is one kind of bacteria and its size is between bacteria and viruses. It's a pathogenic organism and one of its characteristics is that it doesn't have cell walls.
以前は4年に1度くらいの流行がみられましたが，最近ではもう少し頻繁に流行するようです．子どもには多くみられます．
We used to have an epidemic of Mycoplasma Pneumonia about every four years, but recently it has occurred more often. It's common in children.

患者の母: 簡単に移るものなのですか？
Is it contagious?

医師: 咳やくしゃみをした人と一緒にいても移ります．いわゆる飛沫感染ですね．
Yes, it is. If you are with a person who coughs or sneezes, you can become infected. It's called droplet infection.

6. 診断を伝える

患者の母: そうですか．メアリーの症状は重いのでしょうか？
I see. Is Mary's condition serious?

医師: 熱が高いですね．さっき測ったときには，39.5℃ありました．咳もかなり出ていますね．
She has a high fever. Her temperature was 39.5℃ when we took it before. She has a bad cough, too.

患者の母: 治りますか？
Is it curable?

医師: もちろん治りますが，2日ほど入院して点滴を続けた方がいいですね．
Yes, of course! But it's better for her to be hospitalized and get an IV for a couple of days.

患者の母: わかりました．私が付き添った方がいいですか？
OK. Should I accompany her?

医師: そうですね．この病院はもちろん完全看護ですが，おそらくメアリーちゃんが不安がると思うので，できればそうしていただくとよいです．
Yes, I think so. In this hospital, we offer complete nursing care of course, but Mary may feel nervous. So, if possible, it's better if you accompany her.

患者の母: そうします．
I will.

医師: 入院については，受付で説明いたします．入院のしおりもお渡ししますので，ロビーでお待ちください．
Our receptionist will explain the admitting process. She will give you the hospital guide, so please wait in the lobby.

患者の母: ありがとうございます．
Thank you very much.

Part 2　2. 英語で子どもを見る：英語を使った小児科診療・総論

7　薬の説明

　お薬についての説明はとても大切です．

　どんなに正しく診断し，正しく処方しても，的確に説明ができないと効果がないだけではなく，大変な事故につながることもあります．特に，子どもは用量を間違えると大人以上に身体や健康に与える影響が大きいので注意が必要です．

　どのような薬が処方されているのか，何のために薬を飲まなければいけないのかなど服用の意義をキチンと説明することによって，患者さんのコンプライアンスを上げることができるでしょう．

　薬についての説明で，一番気をつけなければならないのは数字です．服薬の説明の中には，「1日3回」とか「1回2錠ずつ」，「3時頃」といろんな数字が出てきます．これらの数字は日本語で説明する場合にもとても注意を払います．英語で説明するときには，紙に書いて渡したり，お薬情報などの用紙に「3 times a day」「2 tablets at one time」「at 3：00 pm」などと書き込んであげたりするのもよい方法でしょう．

　また，服用時を間違えると困る場合もあります．たとえば，利尿薬などは通常午前中に服用するように処方されますが，間違えて夕方や夜に飲んでしまうと，夜中に何度もお手洗いに行かなければならなくなってしまいますし，睡眠導入剤を間違えて日中に飲んでしまうと，眠くなってしまって困ります．

　使い方の説明も重要で，坐薬を飲んでしまったり，シロップ薬を外用薬と間違えて，耳に入れたり，うがいに使ってしまったりという笑い話のようなことも実際に起こっています．

　そして，副作用を説明することも大切です．薬を飲めばだれにでも起こるような軽度なものでも患者さんが心配して飲むのを止めてしまったりすることもあれば，医師の診察を受けなければならないほど重症でも放置してしまうことがあります．起こりうる副作用を説明し，心配しなくてよいものや，すぐに連絡を要するものの区別なども伝えておくと，患者さんも安心して服用できるでしょうね．

　また，薬によっては冷所保存など保管に注意を要するものも少なくありませんし，直射日光や高温を避け，子どもの手が届かないところに保管するということも，一般的ですが大切な注意事項です．

　投薬する時のお薬の状態も日本と外国では違うことがあります．

　例えば日本では，ほとんどの錠剤が1錠ずつPTP包装という形に包装されていますが，外国ではバラの錠剤を瓶に入れて投薬するところも少なくありません．当たり前の事であっても，「包装から取り出して…(take out from the package)」と付け加えましょう．

　また，外国ではシロップ剤や水剤は，スプーンやカップで「何ml量って飲んでください」と説明されることが多いようですが，日本では多くの場合瓶の横の目盛りを使って「1目盛りずつ飲んでください」と指示します．日本語では簡単な説明ですが，英語で説明するのは言い慣れないとむずかしいので，日頃から練習しておくと良いでしょう．もし患者さんから「それは何mlですか？」などという質問があった時には答えられるように準備しておいたり，カップやスプーンを用意してあげたりするのも良いですね．

7．薬の説明

例文

今日は，3種類のお薬が処方されています．	Your doctor prescribed three kinds of medications for you today.
これは，消炎鎮痛薬です．	This is anti-inflammatory medicine.
このお薬は，総合感冒薬です．	This is a general cold remedy.
お薬は，勝手に飲むのを止めないでください．	Please don't stop taking these medications without consulting your doctor.
1日3回，毎食後に2錠ずつ服用してください．	Take two tablets of this medication 3 times a day after each meal.
空腹時に服用してください．	Please take this medicine on an empty stomach.
この糖尿病のお薬は，食事の直前に飲んでください．	Please take this medicine for diabetes just before meals.
この漢方薬は，食間に2包ずつ温かいお湯で飲んでください．	Please take this herbal medicine with hot water between meals.
この抗菌薬は，6時間おきに服用してください．	Please take this antibacterial agent every 6 hours.
この水剤は，ビンの横の1目盛りずつ服用してください．	As for this liquid medication please take one dosage which is equivalent to one measurement as indicated on the side of this bottle.
これは坐薬です．肛門から挿入してください．	This is a suppository. Please insert into the anus.
この解熱薬は，熱が38.5℃以上になったときに飲んでください．	Please take this fever reducer when your temperature goes over 38.5℃.
このお薬を飲むと，眠くなることがあります．車の運転や，機械の操作をする場合には気をつけてください．	You may become drowsy after taking this medicine. Please be careful when you drive a car or operate machinery.
この薬を飲むと，便の色が変わることがあります．	This medication may change the color of your stool.
睡眠導入薬を服用した後は，すぐに床に就いて下さい．	Please go to bed soon after you take a sleeping pill.
軟膏を1日に2回，患部に塗ってください．	Please apply the ointment twice a day to the affected areas.
この経皮吸収パッチ(TTS patch)は，1日に1回貼り替えてください．	Please apply a new TTS patch once a day.
この薬は，直射日光を避けて保管してください．	Please store this medicine away from direct sunlight.
この坐薬は，冷蔵庫など涼しい場所で保管してください．	Please store this suppository in a cool place like a refrigerator.
お薬は，子どもの手が届かないところで保管してください．	Please keep medications out of the reach of children.

> **関連用語**

抗菌薬　antibacterial agent
抗生物質　antibiotic
制酸薬　antacid
胃粘膜保護薬　gastric protective agent
下痢止め　antidiarrhetic, medicine for diarrhea
緩下薬　laxative
吐き気止め　antiemetic, medicine for vomiting
鎮痛薬　analgesic, pain killer
催眠薬　hypnotic agent, narcoleptic, sleeping pill
精神安定薬　tranquilizer
鎮静薬　sedative
血圧降下薬　antihypertensive, high blood pressure medecine
昇圧薬　vasopressor, pressor agent
抗凝固薬　anticoagulant
血栓溶解薬　thrombolytic medicine
脂質異常症治療薬　anti-hyperlipemia, anti-hyperlipidemia
糖尿病薬　anti-diabetic
漢方薬　herbal medicine
血管拡張薬　vasodilator
利尿薬　diuretic, water pill
気管支拡張薬　bronchodilator
去痰薬　expectorant
解熱薬　antipyretic, fever reducer
麻酔薬　anesthetic
リウマチ治療薬　anti-rheumatic agent
咳止め　antitussive, cough medication
吸入薬　inhaler
うがい薬　gargle
かゆみ止め　anti-itch medication
抗ヒスタミン薬　antihistamine
軟膏　ointment
顆粒剤　granular medication
錠剤　pill, tablet
トローチ　lozenge
舌下錠　sublingual medication
水剤　liquid medication

7．薬の説明

初診時の会話例

薬剤師: 今日処方されているお薬を説明します．
I will explain a little about the medication which I will give you today.
今日は，2種類の風邪と感染のお薬が4日分出ていますね．
Today, his/her doctor prescribed two kinds of medications for his/her cold and infection to be taken over four days.

薬剤師: まず，この粉薬は抗菌薬のドライシロップです．
This powder medicine is dry syrup of antibacterial agent.

患者の母: ドライシロップ？
Dry syrup?

薬剤師: はい，このまま飲ませてもいいですし，水に溶いて飲ませてもいいお薬です．
Yes, you can give it as it is or you can dissolve it into water.

患者の母: 味はあるのですか？
Does it have taste?

薬剤師: 甘く味付けがしてあって，イチゴの味がします．
Yes, it's sweetened and tastes like strawberry.
1日に3回1包ずつ，食後に飲ませてください．
Please give him/her one pack of this medication three times a day after each meal.

患者の母: わかりました．
OK.

薬剤師: 食後という指示が出ていますが，もし食事が取れなくても，1日に3回適当な間隔を空けて飲ませてあげてください．
His/Her doctor suggested giving it after meals. But even if he/she can't eat, give him/her three times a day at appropriate intervals.
次に，この水薬は，炎症を抑える薬です．
Next one is a liquid medication for his/her inflammation.
こちらも甘いです．
This is also sweet.
さっきのドライシロップと一緒に1日に3回飲ませてください．
Give him/her this syrup three times a day with the dry syrup.
1回分は，ビンの横のこの目盛りの1目盛りです．
One dosage of this syrup is equal to one division of the scale on the side of this bottle.

患者の母: すみませんが二つの薬の飲み方を紙に書いていただけませんか．
Could you write down how to take these two?

薬剤師: いいですよ．はい，どうぞ．
Sure, here you are.

薬剤師: 坐薬が処方されています．
His/Her doctor prescribed suppositories.

患者の母: それは何のためにですか？
For what?

薬剤師: これは，熱が高くなった時に熱を下げる薬です．
It's a medication to reduce his/her fever when it gets high.

患者の母: どのように使うのですか？
How can I use it?

薬剤師: 熱が38℃以上になったら，この包装から取り出して，お尻から入れてください．
Take out from the wrapping and insert into his/her anus, when his/her body temperature gets 38 degrees Celsius or more.
一度使ったら，次に使用するまでに少なくとも5時間は空けてくださいね．
And please wait for 5 hours at least for the next dose.
使わない時には冷蔵庫で保管しておいてくださいね．
Please keep them in the refrigerator when they are not needed.
ほかに何かお聞きになりたいことはありますか？
Any other questions?

患者の母: 症状がよくなったら，お薬を飲むのを止めてもいいですか？
May I stop taking these medications when his/her symptoms go away?

薬剤師: お薬は勝手に止めないで，かならず主治医に相談して止めてください．
Don't stop taking his/her medications unless advised to do so by his/her doctor.

患者の母: わかりました．
OK, I understand.
それから，ほかのお薬はどこに，またどのように保管しておけばいいですか？
And where and how should I store other two medications?

薬剤師: お子さんの手の届かない，30℃以下の室温で，日光と湿気をさけて保管してください．
Be sure to keep them out of the reach of your children. They should be protected from sunlight and moisture and stored at room temperature below 30 degrees Celsius.
もし，何かいつもと違うような症状に気づかれたら，処方医か薬剤師までご連絡ください．
If you feel anything unusual, please call his/her doctor or your pharmacist.

患者の母 ありがとうございました．
Thank you for your help.

薬剤師 お大事に．
I hope he/she feels better soon.

Column 5

予防接種の回数が多すぎる？

　多くの国では，ワクチン接種の回数は多くても構わないというのが基本方針です．たとえば，NID（National Immunization Day）といって，ワクチン接種の有無にかかわらず，すべての5歳未満児にポリオワクチンの全国一斉投与を行う国や地域もあります．ブラジル，インド，バングラデシュなどでは，定期接種とNIDの両方を律儀に受けた子どもの中には，10回近くポリオワクチンの投与を受けた子どももいます．

　ブラジルから来日したばかりの子どもが，日本の保健センターを受診したときのこと．10回もポリオワクチンの接種をするというのは，きっとワクチンの効果がないからでしょうといわれ，「ぜひ，日本の優秀なワクチンを接種した方がいい」とすすめられたそうです．

　いまや，途上国でも，新しいワクチンがどんどんと導入されています．乳幼児全員を対象としてヒブ（Hib）やB型肝炎を接種している国は少なくありません．5価ワクチンなどの混合ワクチンをルーチンに接種しているアフリカの国もあります．

　外国人の子どもの予防接種の記録をみると，世界の予防接種状況が急速に発展していることがよくわかります．日本も，早く世界標準に追いつきたいですネ．

（中村安秀）

薬の使い方

吸入薬の使い方：inhalant

　子どもに吸入器を使って，薬を投薬する時には，正しくしっかりと吸えているかどうかが問題になります．

　吸入器には，加圧式定量噴霧器（MDI）と粉末噴霧器（DPI）があります．MDIは，容器を押すことによって1回分の薬が強制的に出てくる仕組みですが，DPIは自分の吸う力によって薬を吸うので，吸えているかどうかを確認できない幼い子どもには向いていないといえるでしょう．

　MDIの場合も，子どもは噴霧された薬剤を一度に吸うのは難しいので，スペーサーと呼ばれる補助器具を使います．

①この吸入薬は"スペーサー"を使って吸入することができます．
②使用前に吸入器をよく振ります
③スペーサーに吸入器を正確にセットします
④スペーサーの中に薬を1回分噴霧します
⑤ふつうに息をはきます
⑥スペーサーを口にくわえて，口からゆっくり深く吸います
⑦そのまま息止め（約5秒間）をします
⑧もう一度⑤〜⑦を繰り返します
⑨最後に水でうがいをします
※1回に2噴射以上の処方の場合は，④〜⑧を繰り返し，最後にうがいをします．

①This inhaler is used with a "spacer".
②Before you inhale the medication, shake the inhaler well.
③Insert the inhaler into the spacer firmly.
④Release one dose of the medication into the spacer.
⑤Breathe out normally.
⑥Close lips around spacer and inhale deeply and slowly through your mouth.
⑦Hold your breath for five seconds.
⑧Repeat steps ⑤ to ⑦ again.
⑨Rinse your mouth with water.
※If your dose is more than two puffs at one time, repeat steps ④〜⑧ and rinse your mouth when you finish.

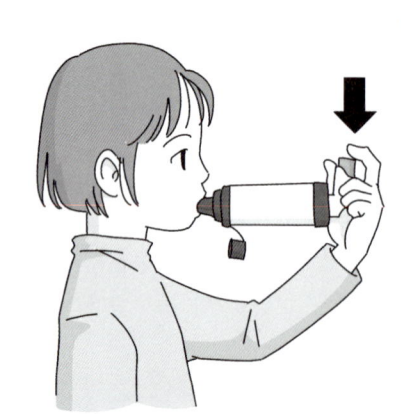

Insert the inhaler into the spacer.

7．薬の説明

坐薬の使い方：suppository

①まず手を洗います．
②薄いビニールの手袋をするか，ラップを人差し指に巻きつけます．
③坐薬を包装から取り出し，水でぬらします．
④子どもを上向きにおむつをかえる時のように寝かせます．
（あるいは，子どもを横向きに寝かせて，膝を曲げさせます．）
⑤片手で坐薬を持ち，もう一方の手でおしりの穴が見えるまでお尻を開きます．
⑥ゆっくりと坐薬をおしりの穴に挿入し，見えなくなるまで入ったら人差し指を入れて少し押し，確実に挿入されて出てこないかどうかを確かめます．
⑦入れ終わったら2～3分間，肛門を抑えて静かにしています．

①Wash your hands thoroughly.
②Put on plastic gloves or cover your index finger with plastic wrap.
③Remove plastic wrap from the suppository and wet the suppository with water.
④Lay your child on his/her back and raise his/her legs as if to change a diaper.
(or Lay your child on either side and bend his/her knees toward the chest.)
⑤Hold the suppository with one hand and open the buttocks with the other until you can see the anus.
⑥Gently insert the suppository into the anus until it disappears. Make sure the suppository is completely inside the rectum by using the tip of your index finger.
⑦Press the anus gently for a couple of minutes to keep the suppository inside.

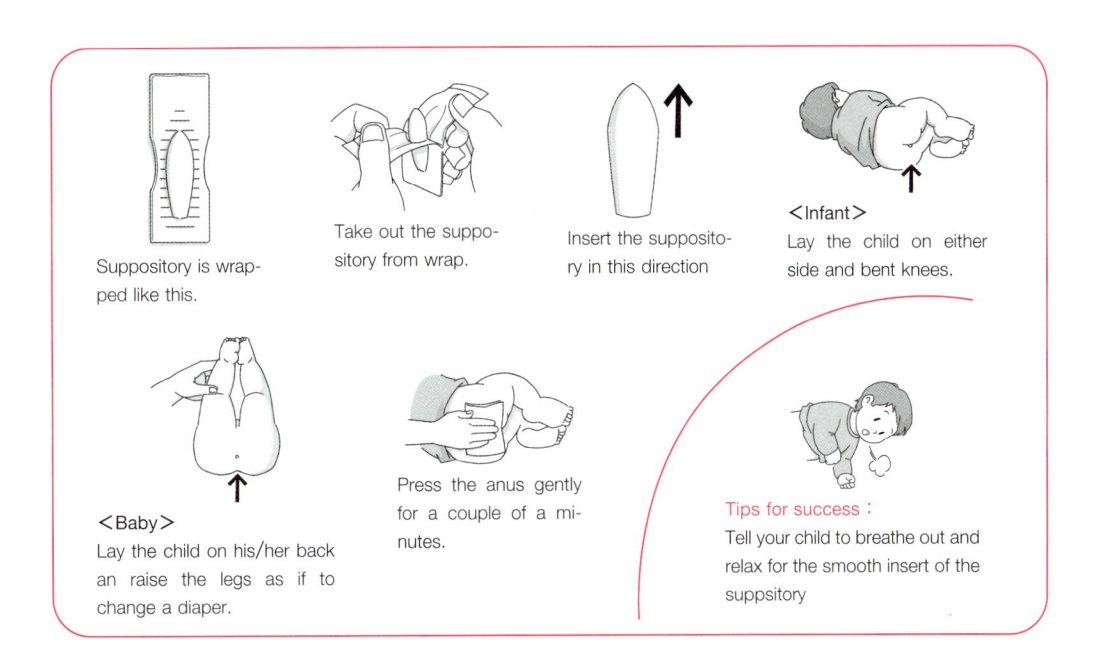

Suppository is wrapped like this.

Take out the suppository from wrap.

Insert the suppository in this direction

<Infant>
Lay the child on either side and bent knees.

<Baby>
Lay the child on his/her back an raise the legs as if to change a diaper.

Press the anus gently for a couple of a minutes.

Tips for success：
Tell your child to breathe out and relax for the smooth insert of the suppsitory

目薬の使い方：eye drops

①子どもの顔（特に目の周辺）が汚れていないかチェックし，もし汚れているなら洗うか，ぬれたタオルで拭きましょう．

②次に自分の手もきれいに洗い，タオルで拭きます．

③子どもを上向きに寝かせるか，頭を後ろに倒します．

④目を閉じさせます．

⑤自分の指で，静かに目を開けます．

⑥目薬の容器の先端が目に触れないようにして，薬を目頭に1滴差します．

⑦5秒から10秒間くらい目を閉じたままにして，あふれた薬液はきれいな紙で拭き取ります．

①Check if your child's face is clean. If not, wash or wipe it with wet towel.

②Next, wash your hands thoroughly and dry with a towel.

③Lay your child on his/her back, or tilt his/her head back.

④Have your child close his/her eyes.

⑤Gently opten the affected eye with your fingers.

⑥Apply the eye drops into the inner corner of the eyes without touching the tip of the eye dropper to the surface of the eye.

⑦Have your child keep his/her eyes closed for 5 to 10 seconds. Wipe away any excess eye drops with clean tissue.

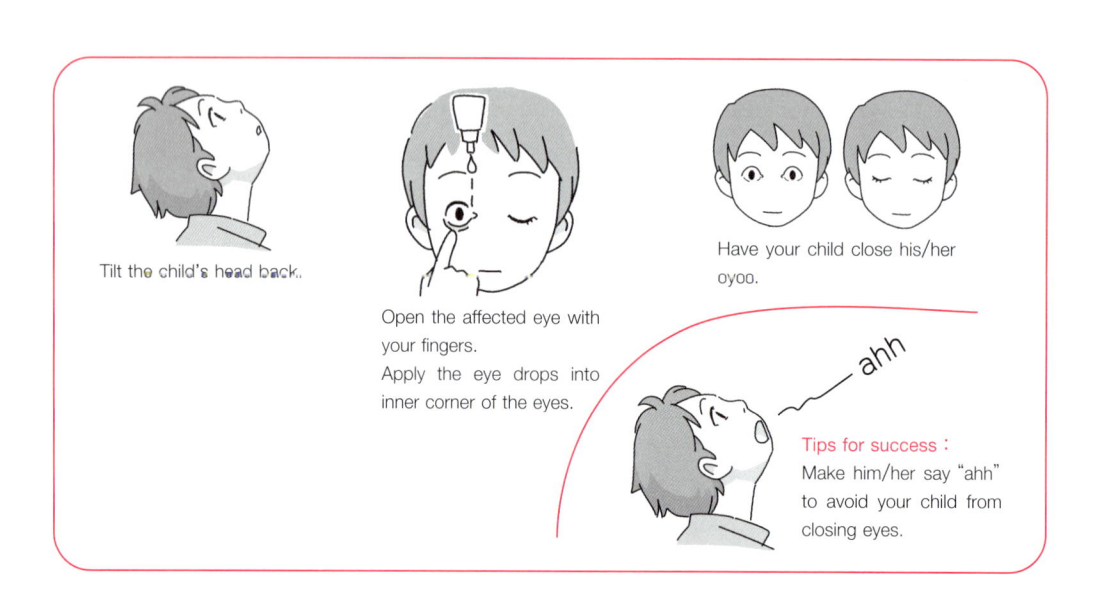

Tilt the child's head back.

Open the affected eye with your fingers.
Apply the eye drops into inner corner of the eyes.

Have your child close his/her oyoo.

Tips for success：
Make him/her say "ahh" to avoid your child from closing eyes.

7．薬の説明

塗り薬の塗り方：ointment, liniment

①まず，自分の手を洗い，タオルでよく乾かします．

②次に，必要量の軟膏を人差し指で取ります．

※軟膏の量は人差し指で量ることができます．標準的な5mmのノズルのチューブの場合，人差し指の先から第1関節までの長さの量（1FTU）でおおよそ両手のひらの面積を塗ることができます．

③指の腹や手のひらを使って，やさしくゆっくりと軟膏（クリーム）が見えなくなるまでのばして下さい．

④通常，薄く塗るだけで十分です．

⑤塗り終わったら，手を洗いましょう．

①First, wash your hands thoroughly and dry completely with a towel.

②Next, take the needed amount of ointment (cream) with using your index finger.

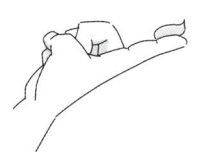

※You can measure the amount of the needed ointment (cream) by fingertip units (FTU). One FTU is the amount of ointment (cream) that reaches from the tip to the first crease of the index finger when squeezed from a tube with a standard 5mm nozzle.

One FTU is usually enough to cover an area about twice the size of an adult's hand.

③Gently spread the ointment (cream) across the affected area little by little, rubbing it in slowly until the ointment (cream) has disappeared.

④A thin layer is usually sufficient.

⑤Wash your hands again when done.

You can measure the amount of the needed ointment (cream) by fingertip units (FTU).

As for lotion, you can measure by 1 Yen coin.

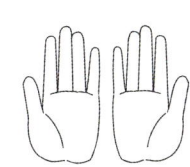

1 FTU is enough to spread out the area of skin twice the size of the palm of adult's hand.

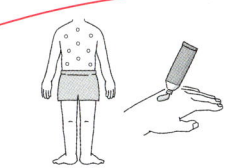

Tips for success：
If you have to cover a wide area, you should place ointment/cream in several spots first, and then spread it over.

内服薬の飲ませ方：internal medicine

内服薬には，粉薬，顆粒，ドライシロップ，錠剤，カプセル，シロップなどがあります．

一般的に5歳をすぎると錠剤やカプセルが飲めるようになるとされていますが，もしまだ飲めないような場合には，医師や薬剤師に伝えましょう．小児に使われるお薬にはほとんど，粉薬やドライシロップといって甘く味付けした剤形があります．

また，錠剤を割ったりつぶしたり，あるいはカプセルをはずして飲ませたりする場合には，必ず薬剤師に相談してください．お薬の中には，割ったり，カプセルをはずしたりすることによって，作用が強く出すぎたり，早く吸収されたり，あるいは苦味が出てしまったりすることがあります．

【赤ちゃんに薬を飲ませるコツ　Tips to give your baby medications】

●粉薬　Powdered medication

①粉薬は少しの水か白湯でペースト状に練り，頬の内側に塗りつけます．そして，すぐに白湯を飲ませて，飲み込ませます．果汁などを飲める場合には，お水の代わりに果汁で混ぜてもよいでしょう．（処方したお医者さんに聞いてください．）

①Add a little bit of water or boild water to the powder to make a paste.
Put it inside your baby's cheek and immediately give him/her some water so that he/she will swallow the medication.
If he/she can drink juice, you can use juice instead of water.（Ask his/her doctor first.）

②少しの水や白湯で溶かし哺乳瓶やスポイトを使って飲ませることもできますが，飲み残しがないように飲みきれる量の水か白湯に溶かすように注意してください．

②You can use a bottle or a plastic syringe to give the medication after dissolving it with a small amount of water or boild water, but make sure that your baby can finish the complete dose.

③スプーンが使えるようになっていたら，少しのヨーグルトや好きなゼリーに混ぜて，与えてもよいでしょう．

③If your baby can eat with a spoon, you can mix the medication with a small amount of yogurt or his/her favorite jelly.

●シロップ（水薬）Syrup（liquid medicine）

①スポイトに1回分のお薬を取り，口の端から口の中に入れて，飲ませます．口の真ん中から入れると，気管に入ったりむせたりするので，気をつけましょう．すぐ後に，白湯を飲ませて，お薬をのみこませます．

①Draw the prescribed amount of syrup into the plastic syringe and place the end of the syringe in a corner of your baby's mouth, not in the center where it might cause your baby to choke.
Squeeze out the medication into your baby's mouth and give him/her some water to wash it down.

7．薬の説明

②哺乳瓶に入れて飲ませることもできます．少しの水か白湯などで薄めてもよいですが，飲みきれる量にするように注意して下さい．

③スプーンで少しずつ飲ませることもできます．口からあふれないように，一匙にたくさん入れすぎないように気をつけましょう．

②A baby bottle can also be used to give the medication. You may dilute the medication with water or boild water, but make sure that your baby can finish the completely dose.

③You can give liquid medication using a spoon. Be careful not to give too much at one time, in order to avoid the medicine spilling out from his/her mouth.

＜Powdered medication＞

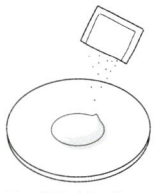

Add a little bit of water to the powdered medication to make a paste.

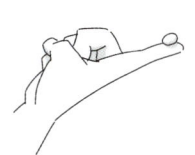

Put it inside the cheek and give him/her water soon to swallow.

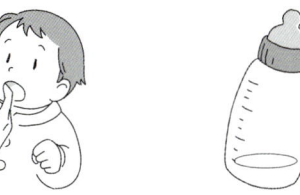

You can use a bottle after mixing the medication with water, but make sure that your baby can finish the complete dose.

＜Syrup (liquid medicine)＞

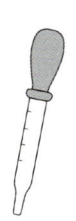

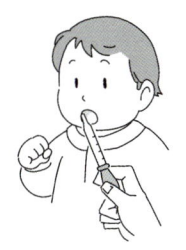

Draw the prescribed amount of syrup into the syringe.
Place the syringe in a corner of your baby's mouth.

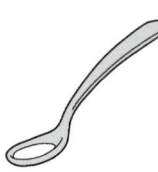

You can give liquid medicine using a spoon. Be careful not to put too much medicine at one time.

食後と食前：After and before meals

① 「食後」とは，食事の後 30 分以内を指しますが，時間が経つと忘れてしまうこともあるので，とくに指示がない限りは，食後すぐに飲んでも大丈夫です．

② また，「食前」は，食事の前 30 分以内を指します．

③ 「食後」と指示される薬が多いですが，糖尿病の薬などで，必ず「食前」に服用しなければならない薬もあります．

④ 赤ちゃんの場合には，おなかがいっぱいだと薬を飲んでくれないことが多いので，おなかが空いている時の方が飲ませやすいでしょう．

⑤ また，嫌がって激しく泣いているような時には，無理に飲ませると気管に入ってしまうことがあり危険なので，一旦休んで，機嫌が良くなってから再度飲ませてみてください．

① "After meals" means within 30 minutes of eating. However, you can take medications immediately after eating in order to avoid forgetting unless you are especialy told by a physician or a pharmacist to wait 30 minutes.

② "Before meals" means within 30 minutes before eating.

③ Many medications are prescribed to take after meals, but there are some medications which should always be taken before meals. (e.g. medications for diabetes mellitus)

④ Babies often refuse medications when they are full.
They are more likely to accept medication when they are hungry.
Therefore, give the medication before meals unless instructed otherwise by a physician or a pharmacist.

⑤ In addition, never try to give a medication to a crying baby. When the baby is crying, there is the risk that he/she will choke on the medication. If your baby rejects a medication and starts crying, wait a while until he/she has calmed down before trying again.

8 会計時のトラブルをさけるために

　診察や検査が終わると，最後にお金を払って帰りますが，医療機関のシステムによっては，ここで次の予約を取ったり，また最近では処方せんを発行したりするところも増えてきました．会計の受付での会話も多様になってきたので，備えておくと安心です．

　日本の医療機関でも最近はクレジットカードで支払えるところが出てきましたが，まだまだ少ないようですね．「クレジットカードで支払えますか？」とか「クレジットカードを使えますか？」と聞く時には，「私」を主語にする場合には，「Can I use a credit card?」のように「use」を使い，「あなた（医療機関）」を主語にする場合には「Do you accept a credit card?」のように「accept」を使います．

　外国からの患者さんの場合には，医療保険にも色々な種類があり，一旦全額を支払ってもらってから後で還付されるものも多いので，説明ができるようにしておくとトラブルが少ないでしょう．また，「医療保険に入っている」は「be covered by health insurance」のように「cover」を使います．

　医療にかかる費用の設定の違いも多く，たとえば日本では診断書や処方箋を発行するのに費用がかかりますが，外国ではかからない国が多いので，何の費用なのかを説明できるようにしておくといいですね．

　「予約」という意味の英語はいろいろありますが，診察の予約は「appointment」を使います．ですから，「○○先生に次回診察の予約を取る」という時には，「make an appointment to see Dr. ○○．」のようになります．また「make」の代わりに「schedule」と言ってもよいでしょう．

　最近は，処方された薬を院外の薬局で受け取る事が増えました．この場合は処方せんが発行されるのですが，「処方せんを発行する」というのは「issue a prescription」と言います．受付で「処方せんが発行されていますよ．」という場合には「あなた」を主語にして「You have a prescription.」と言ってもよいでしょう．

　院外処方せんを発行している医療機関では，薬局にファックスを送るサービスをすることもあります．「fax」という単語は，「send a fax」あるいは「send by fax」などのように名詞として，あるいは「ファックスを送る」という動詞としても使えます．

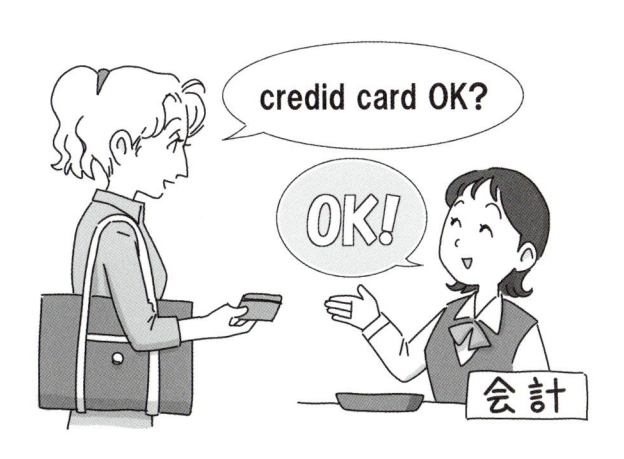

例文

クレジットカードで支払えますか？	・Do you accept a credit card? ・Can I pay by credit card? ・Can I pay with a credit card?
申し訳ありませんが，クレジットカードではお支払いいただけません．	・I'm sorry but we do not accept any credit cards. ・I'm afraid we do not accept any credit cards.
現金でお支払いください．	・Please pay by cash. ・We accept only cash.
医療保険に入っていない場合には，全額自費払いになります．	If you are not covered by any health insurance, you have to pay your medical fee at your own expenses.
合計で 2,350 円になります．	Today's medical fee comes to a total of 2350 yen.
おつりは，7,650 円です．	Here is your change of 7,650 yen.
こちらが本日の診療明細書です．	This is the detailed statement of today's services.
領収書です．	Here is the receipt.
診療費には，診察代，検査費用と処方せん発行手数料が含まれています．	Your bill includes the doctor's fee, lab fees and a fee for issuing the prescription.
医療費は国民健康保険で7割が支払われ，残り3割を自己負担していただきます．	70% of your medical fee is covered by national health insurance and the rest is your co-payment.
一旦全額をお支払いいただいて，後からご加入の保険会社に請求後，そちらの方から還付されます．	After you pay the total fee, send in a claim to your insurance company and they will reimburse you.
10月18日以降でご都合の良い日に予約をお取りします．	We will schedule your next appointment after October 18th.
もし急にご都合が悪くなり，お越しいただけない時にはお電話ください．	If for some reason you are unable to come, please call to let us know.
次の診察予約日までに急な病状の変化がありましたら，いつでもご連絡ください．	If you have any changes to your condition, please contact us.
お薬が処方されていますので，隣の窓口で処方せんを受け取ってください．	Your doctor prescribed some medications. Please get your prescription at the next window.
これは院外処方せんですので，保険調剤薬局でお薬を受け取ってください．	This is your prescription. Please get your medications at any pharmacy.
お薬はどこの薬局でも受け取ることができますが，もしかかりつけの薬局がありましたら，こちらからファックスをお送りすることもできます．	You can get your medications at any pharmacy. However, if you have a regular pharmacy, we can send your prescription by fax there.

8. 会計時のトラブルをさけるために

関連用語

（クレジットカードなどに）対応している　accept
合計で　in total
おつり　change
診療明細書　detailed statement of services
国民健康保険　national health insurance
自己負担　co-payment, deductible fee
自費で　at your own expense
還付する　reimburse
予約　appointment
処方せん　prescription
薬局　pharmacy
かかりつけの薬局　regular pharmacy

Column 6

医療費の支払い方法―病院で使える⁉クレジットカード―

　ラテン語の Hospes が語源となっているホテル（Hotel）と病院（Hospital）．日本では，多くのホテルでクレジットカードが使用できるのに，病院ではクレジットカードが使えなかったなんて話は聞きませんか？

　病院を受診し診察を受けた後には，必ず医療費の支払いがあります．外国人の旅行者から，診察前に，自費では医療費がいくらぐらいかかるか，クレジットカードが使用できるかどうか質問されることがよくあります．

　海外の private hospital では，大抵クレジットカードでの支払いが可能です．しかし，以前，日本の病院ではクレジットカードが使えないなんてことがありました．でも，最近は日本でも，国立病院や労災病院が 2004 年からクレジットカードによる医療費支払いが可能になるなど，導入が検討されている病院も増えてはきています．

　もちろん，日本人でもクレジットカードでの支払いを希望される方が多く，この流れは増してくることでしょう．利用する方からすれば，便利であることと，クレジットカードのポイントがつくことも魅力です．逆に，クレジットカードが使用できることで，医療費の未払いが減ったという病院のメリットもあるようです．

（福島慎二）

初診時の会話例

受付: 今日の診療費は，合計で 2,350 円です。
Today's medical fee comes to a total of 2,350 yen.

患者の母: 医療保険を使っての金額ですか？
Is this a deductible fee?

受付: はい，そうです。
医療費の 7 割が入っていらっしゃる国民健康保険で支払われ，残りの 3 割が自己負担になります。
Yes, it is.
70% of the medical fee is covered by national health insurance and you need to pay the rest of 30% as co-payment.

患者の母: わかりました。
I see.

受付: 次回のご予約ですが，10 月 18 日以降で取ることができます。
We can schedule your next appointment after October 18th.

患者の母: では，10 月 18 日にお願いします。
Then, please make my appointment on October 18th.

受付: わかりました。
もし，次回予約日までに急な病状の変化が見られましたら，すぐにご連絡ください。
All right.
If your child's condition gets worse by his/her next appointment, please contact us.

患者の母: ありがとうございます。
Thank you.

受付: また，もし何かのご都合でその日に来られない場合にも，お電話ください。
Also, if for some reason he/she is unable to come, please call to let us know.

患者の母: わかりました。そうします。
OK. I will.

8．会計時のトラブルをさけるために

受付： 今日はお薬も処方されています．当院では，院外処方せんをお出ししていますので，保険調剤薬局でお薬をもらってください．
お薬はどこの薬局でも受け取ることができますが，もしかかりつけの薬局がありましたら，こちらからファックスをお送りすることもできます．
Your child's doctor prescribed some medications. Our clinic issues a prescription. So, please get the medication at a pharmacy that takes his/her health insurance.
You can get the medications at any pharmacy, but if you have a regular pharmacy, we can send his/her prescription by fax to the pharmacy.

患者の母： ファックスを送れば，何かメリットはありますか？
Is there any benefit to faxing it?

受付： スミスさんが薬局に行くまでに，お薬を用意してくれますので，待ち時間が短くなりますね．
Usually, when we send a fax, the pharmacies fill your child's prescription before you get there. It will decrease your wait time.

患者の母： まあ！それは助かります．では，栄町のさくら薬局にしてください．
Wow! That's a real help! Then please fax it to Sakura Pharmacy in Sakae-machi.

受付： わかりました．すぐにお送りします．
Yes, ma'am.
We will send it immediately.

患者の母： ありがとうございました．
Thank you very much!

受付： どういたしまして．お大事に．
You are welcome.
Please take care!

3章

症状を英語で把握する
（英語を使った小児科診療・各論）

To understand the patient's symptom

The aim of this chapter

患者から症状を聞き取る際の質問集.

☝があるところは，答えを指さしで指示してもらい，☑印のところは✓をして説明したり，症状を✓してもらって答えを引き出せるようになっています.

Part 3　3. 症状を英語で把握する：英語を使った小児科診療・各論

1 基本的な問診
Basic intake questionnaire

●個人情報を聴取する Personal data

お子さんのお名前	生年月日
Name of Child	Birth Date: Year, Month, Day

性別	住所・電話番号
Sex	Address・Phone number

●基本的な問診　Basic intake questionnaire

1. どんな症状がありますか？
   What kind of symptom does your child have?
   - ☐ 発熱　Has a fever
   - ☐ 元気がない　Lacks energy
   - ☐ 機嫌が悪い　Is in a bad mood
   - ☐ 食欲不振　Has little appetite
   - ☐ 咳　Has a cough
   - ☐ 鼻水　Has a runny nose
   - ☐ のどが痛い　Has a sore throat
   - ☐ 嘔吐　Has been vomiting, throwing-up
   - ☐ 吐き気　Has nausea
   - ☐ 下痢　Has diarrhea
   - ☐ 便秘　Has constipation, is constipated
   - ☐ 頭痛　Has a headache
   - ☐ 腹痛　Has abdominal pain (stomachache)
   - ☐ 胸痛　Has chest pain
   - ☐ むくみ　Has Swelling
   - ☐ 発疹　Has a rash
   - ☐ ひきつけ　Has seizures
   - ☐ その他　Other

2. いま，飲んでいる薬はありますか？
   Are you currently taking medication?

3. 妊娠中，出産の状態を教えてください．
   Would you describe your pregnancy and delivery?
   - ■ 妊娠中の経過は，順調でしたか？
     Did the course of your pregnancy go well?
   - ■ 妊娠何週目で，出産しましたか？
     At what week was your child born?

1．基本的な問診　Basic intake questionnaire

■出産は，正常分娩でしたか？
　Was that delivery normal?
■出生時の赤ちゃんの体重は何グラムでしたか？
　How much was your baby's weight at birth?
■出産時に，お母さんは何歳でしたか？
　How old were you when you gave birth?

4．過去に，どのような病気をしましたか？
　　Has your child ever had any of the following illnesses?
　□麻疹（はしか）　Measles
　□風疹　Rubella
　□水ぼうそう　Varicella, Chickenpox
　□おたふくかぜ　Mumps
　□アトピー性皮膚炎　Atopic dermatitis
　□気管支ぜんそく　Bronchial asthma
　□熱性けいれん　Febrile seizures
　□その他の病気　Other illnesses

■過去に，入院したことがありますか？
　Has your child ever been hospitalized?
　■どんな病気でしたか？
　　What was the reason of the hospitalization?
　■そのエピソードは，いつのことですか？
　　When did your child have this episode?
　■何日間，入院しましたか？
　　How many days was your child hospitalized?
■過去に，手術したことがありますか？
　Has your child undergone a surgery?
　■それは，どんな病気でしたか？
　　What was the reason?
　■そのエピソードは，いつのことですか？
　　When did your child have this episode?

5．食べ物や薬などで，アレルギーを生じたことがありますか？
　　Have you ever been allergic to food or medication?
　　（アレルギーの原因となる薬や食べものなどは，次ページのMemoを参考にして下さい．）

6．すでに受けた予防接種を教えてください．
　　Let us know which of the following vaccinations your child has received?
　□BCG　BCG vaccination
　□三種混合　DPT：Diphtheria, Pertussis, Tetanus
　□ポリオ　Polio vaccination
　□麻疹・風疹　MR：Measles, Rubella

55

- ☐ 麻疹・風疹・おたふくかぜ　MMR：Measles, Mumps, Rubella
- ☐ 水ぼうそう　Varicella, Chickenpox
- ☐ ヒブ　Hib：Haemophilus influenzae type B
- ☐ インフルエンザ　Influenza
- ☐ B 型肝炎　Hepatitis B
- ☐ 肺炎球菌　Pneumococcal
- ☐ ロタウイルス　Rotavirus
- ☐ A 型肝炎　Hepatitis A
- ☐ その他　Other

7．お子さんは健康保険をもっていますか？
　　Does your child have medical insurance?

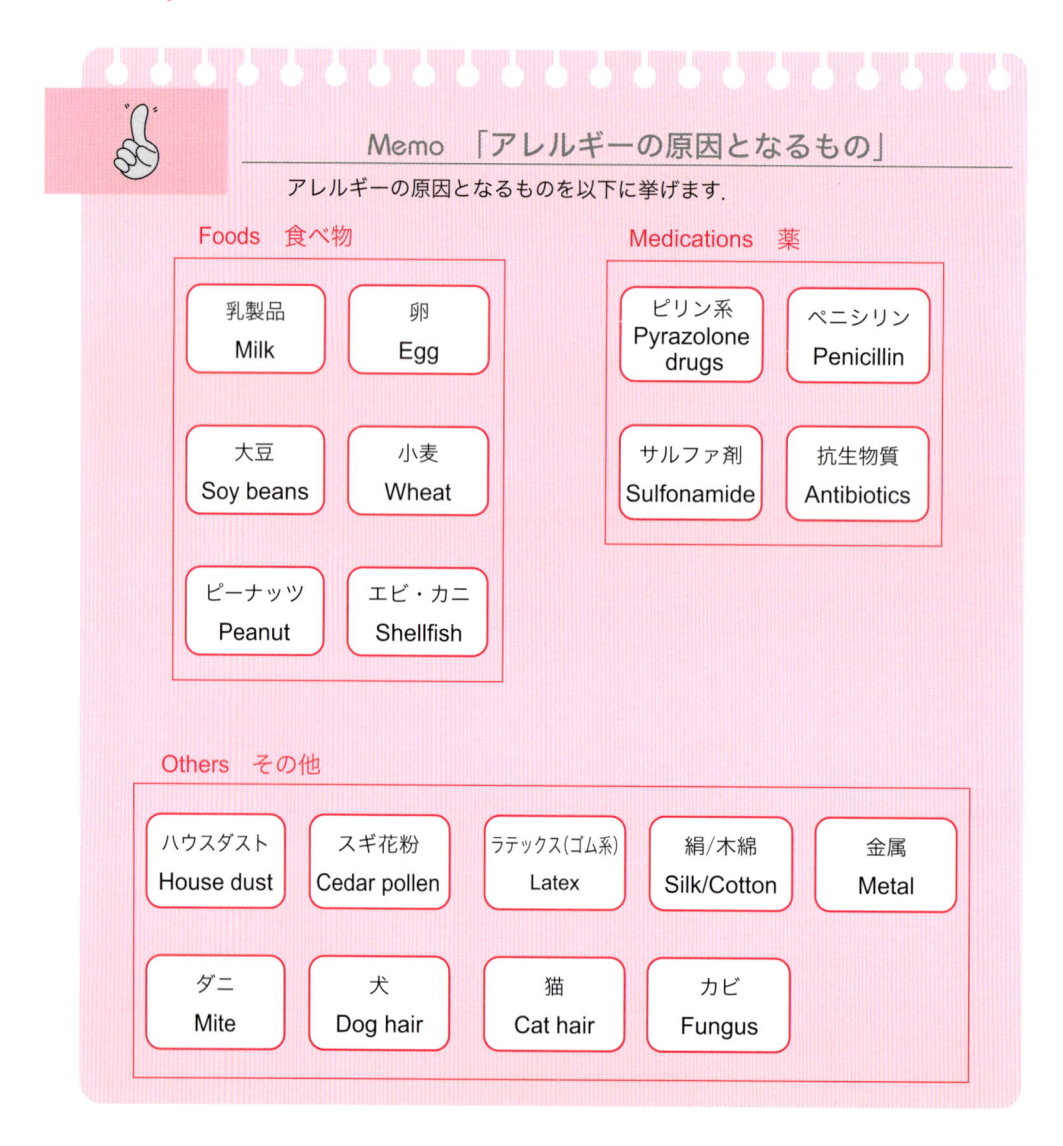

Memo 「アレルギーの原因となるもの」

アレルギーの原因となるものを以下に挙げます．

Foods　食べ物

乳製品 Milk	卵 Egg
大豆 Soy beans	小麦 Wheat
ピーナッツ Peanut	エビ・カニ Shellfish

Medications　薬

ピリン系 Pyrazolone drugs	ペニシリン Penicillin
サルファ剤 Sulfonamide	抗生物質 Antibiotics

Others　その他

ハウスダスト House dust	スギ花粉 Cedar pollen	ラテックス(ゴム系) Latex	絹/木綿 Silk/Cotton	金属 Metal
ダニ Mite	犬 Dog hair	猫 Cat hair	カビ Fungus	

Part 3　3. 症状を英語で把握する：英語を使った小児科診療・各論

2 健　診
Health check-up for your baby/child

場面別
問診
健診
栄養
検査
診断

●個人情報を聴取する Personal data

お子さんのお名前	生年月日
Name of Child	Birth Date: Year, Month, Day

性別	住所・電話番号
Sex	Address・Phone number

●健　診　Health check-up

1. 新生児期
Newborn Phase

■赤ちゃんに初めてお乳を飲ませたのは生後何時間たってからですか？
At how many hours after delivery did you first feed your baby?

■そのとき，与えたお乳は母乳ですか？　人工乳ですか？
Was it breastfeeding or formula?

■先天性代謝異常等検査を受けましたか？
Was your baby checked for congenital metabolic diseases?
（とくに，海外で出産した場合には，必ずこの質問をしてください．
なお，国によっては，検査項目が日本よりも少ないことがあります．）

■いま，赤ちゃんは，お乳をよく飲みますか？
Does your baby suck well now?

■いま，赤ちゃんは，1日に何回くらいウンチをしますか？
How many times does your baby have a bowel movement each day?

2. 1か月健診
One Month Medical Health Check-up

■裸にすると手足をよく動かしますか？
Does your baby actively move his/her legs and arms when being undressed or dressed?

■赤ちゃんは，お乳をよく飲みますか？
Does your baby suck well?

■大きな音にビクッと手足を伸ばしたり，泣き出すことがありますか？
Does your baby move his/her arms and legs or start to cry in response to a loud noise or sound?

　■これはモロー反射（Moro Reflex）といいます．
　This is called Moro Reflex.

　■赤ちゃんにみられる正常反射の一つです．
　This is one of normal reflex seen commonly in babies.

　■4か月ごろまでに，消えていきます．
　This will disappear by the fourth month.

57

■赤ちゃんのおへそはかわいていますか？
　Is your baby's navel dry?
■うすい黄色，クリーム色，灰白色の便が続いていますか？
　Has your baby been having bowel movements in light yellow, cream or grayish color?

3．3〜4か月健診
Health Check-up for your baby at three to four months old
■首がすわりましたか？
　Does your baby hold his/her head upright?
■あやすとよく笑いますか？
　Does your baby laugh or smile when he/she is touched or held?
■見えない方向から声をかけてみると，そちらの方を見ようとしますか？
　Does your baby try to look toward the direction of your voices when you call him/her from a place out of his/her sight?
■目つきや目の動きがおかしいのではないかと気になりますか？
　Do you find anything unusual in your baby's eye expressions or movements?
■いま赤ちゃんに与えているお乳は母乳ですか？　人工乳ですか？　両方ですか？
　Are you breastfeeding or giving formula or both?

4．6〜7か月健診
Health check-up for your baby at six to seven months old
■寝返りをしますか？
　Does your baby turn over?
■おすわりをしますか？
　Does your baby sit up by himself/herself without support?

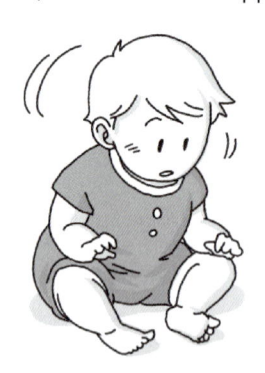

■からだのそばにあるおもちゃに手をのばしてつかみますか？
　Does your baby reach out for toys near him/her?
■家族といっしょにいるとき，話しかけるような声を出しますか？
　Does your baby babble when he/she is with his/her family?
■テレビやラジオの音がしはじめると，すぐそちらを見ますか？
　Does your baby turn his/her head toward the TV or radio when it is on?
■いつごろから，離乳食を始めましたか？
　At what age, did you start to feed solid foods to your baby?

2. 健 診　Health check-up for your baby/child

5．9〜10か月健診
Health check-up for your baby at nine to ten months

- はいはいをしますか？
  Does your baby crawl?
- つかまり立ちができますか？
  Does your baby pull him/herself up?
- 指で，小さい物をつまみますか？
  Does your baby pick up small objects with his/her fingers?
- 機嫌よくひとりで遊んでいることがありますか？
  Does your baby play by himself/herself?
- そっと近づいて，ささやき声で呼びかけると，振り向きますか？
  Does your baby turn around when you come softly and whisper to him/her?
- 歯が生えてきましたか？
  Has your baby cut his/her first tooth?

6．1歳健診
Health check-up for your baby at one year old

- つたい歩きをしますか？
  Has your baby started to walk by holding on something for support?
- バイバイ，コンニチワなどの身振りをしますか？
  Does your baby wave his/her hand goodbye or greet you?
- テレビなどの音楽に合わせて，からだを楽しそうに動かしますか？
  Does your baby sway pleasantly to the music from TV or others?
- 大人のいう簡単なことばがわかりますか？
  たとえば，おいで，ちょうだいなどのことばです．
  Does your baby understand such simple words as "Come here" or "Give it to me".
- 相手になって遊んであげると喜びますか？
  Does your baby seem to enjoy playing with you?
- 歯は何本，生えていますか？
  How many teeth does your baby have now?

7．1歳6か月健診
Health check-up for your baby at eighteen months old

- ひとりで上手に歩きますか？
  Does your baby walk well on his/her own?
- ひとり歩きができるようになったのは，いつですか？
  When did your baby start to walk by himself/herself?
- ママ，ブーブーなど意味のあることばを話しますか？
  Does your baby utter meaningful words such as "mama" or "papa"?
  - どんな単語を話しますか？
- 自分でコップを持って水を飲めますか？
  Can your baby drink water from a cup by himself/herself?

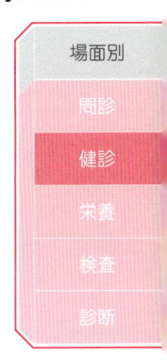

■哺乳ビンを使っていますか？
　Is your baby drinking from a bottle?
■極端にまぶしがったり，目の動きがおかしいと気になりますか？
　Do you find your baby being too sensitive to light or having unusual eye movements?
■テレビを見るとき目を細めたり，首を傾けたりしますか？
　Does your baby watch TV with his/her eyes half-closed or by inclining his/her head?
■うしろから名前を呼んだとき，振り向きますか？
　Does your baby look back when you call him/her from behind?
■どんな遊びが好きですか？
　What kind of activities does your baby like to do?
■歯は何本，生えていますか？
　How many teeth does your child have?

8．3歳健診
Health check-up for your child at three years old

■自分の名前が言えますか？
　Can your child say his/her name?
■歯みがきや手洗いをしていますか？
　Does your child brush his/her teeth and wash his/her hands?
■斜視はありますか？
　Does your child appear to be cross-eyed?
■物を見るとき目を細めたり，極端に近づけて見たりしますか？
　Does your child squint at an object or move extremely close to see something?
■耳の聞こえが悪いのではないかと気になりますか？
　Does your child seem to suffer from hearing loss?
■遊び友だちがいますか？
　Does your child have friends to play with?

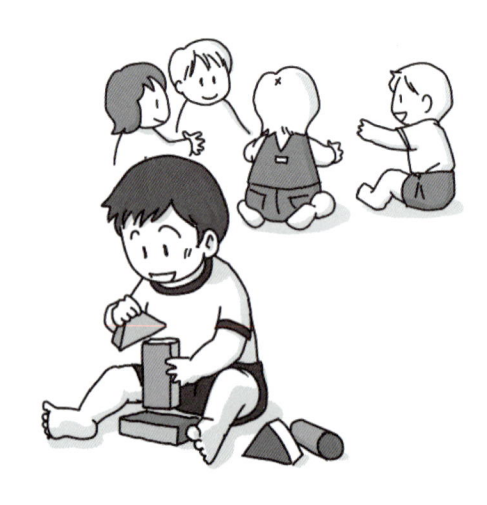

2．健　診　Health check-up for your baby/child

9．4歳健診
Health check-up for your child at four years old

■ 衣服の着脱がひとりでできますか？
Does your child take off or put on his/her clothes on his/her own?

■ 友だちといっしょに遊んでいますか？
Does your child play with his/her friends?

■ 食事の前に，手を洗っていますか？
Does your child wash his/her hands before meals?

■ おしっこをひとりでしますか？
Does your child go to the toilet and urinate by him/herself?

■ 子育てについて困難を感じることはありますか？
Have you ever had trouble with your child-rearing?

10．5歳健診
Health check-up for your child at five years old

■ 赤，黄，緑，青などの色がわかりますか？
Does your child identify colors such as red, yellow, green and blue?

■ 動物や花をかわいがったりしていますか？
Does your child care for animals and flowers?

■ 大便をひとりでしますか？
Does your child go to toilet and empty his/her bowels?

■ 歯みがきをしていますか？
Does your child wash his/her teeth?

■ 子育てについて困難を感じることはありますか？
Have you ever had trouble with your child-rearing?

ポイント

❶ 健診では，子どもの成長と発達をチェックするだけでなく，ちょっとした気がかりなどを相談できる絶好の場です．保護者から質問しやすいように，「何か質問はありませんか？（Do you have any questions?）」と，こちらから聞いてあげることも大切です．

❷ 育児に対して自信がない，子どもの育て方で迷っている，という育児不安をもつ保護者は少なくありません．まず，保護者の悩みを傾聴してから，助言をしてあげてください．

❸ 育児は文化です．外国人の母親の多くは，母国の育児と日本の育児の違いにとまどっています．私は，母親の出身国の文化を尊重した上で，日本のやり方を押し付けるのではなく，日本の育児方法を知識として提供するというスタンスをとっています．

Part 3 3．症状を英語で把握する：英語を使った小児科診療・各論

3 栄養方法
Nutrition chart

● 個人情報を聴取する Personal data

お子さんのお名前	生年月日
Name of Child	Birth Date: Year, Month, Day

性別	住所・電話番号
Sex	Address・Phone number

● 栄養方法　Nutrition chart

1．栄養に関する質問
   Questions related to nutrition
   ■母乳をよく飲んでいますか？
   Does your baby suck well at the breast?
   ■1日に何回，離乳食をあげていますか？
   How many times a day do you give baby food to your baby?
   ■離乳食は手づくりしていますか？　それとも，市販のものを使っていますか？
   Do you make your baby food? Or do you feed store-bought baby food?
   ■離乳食をよく食べますか？
   Does your baby like to eat baby food?
   ■好きな食べ物は何ですか？
   What kind of food does your child/baby like most?
   ■嫌いな食べ物は何ですか？
   What kind of food does your child/baby not like to eat?
   ■どんなおやつをあげていますか？
   What kind of snack do you give to your child/baby?

2．食事に関する質問
   Questions related to meal
   ■食事のとき，誰といっしょに食べていますか？
   Who stays with your child/baby when he/she eats?
   ■スプーンを使って食事していますか？
   Does your child/baby use a spoon to eat?
   ■お箸を使えるようになりましたか？
   Has your child used chopsticks?

3．栄養方法　Nutrition chart

Memo 「日本の離乳食ガイドライン」

日本の離乳食ガイドラインは以下の通りです．

離乳食の進め方の目安（日本の離乳食ガイドライン）
Solid Foods Chart Table

	離乳初期 Introductory Stage	離乳中期 First Stage	離乳後期 Second Stage	離乳完了期 Final Stage
月齢（か月） Month Age	5〜6か月 5-6 Months	7〜8か月 7-8 Months	9〜11か月 9-11 Months	12〜15か月 12-15 Months
調理形態 Texture of Solids	ドロドロ状 Soft, pureed and strained	舌でつぶせる固さ Pureed and strained	歯ぐきでつぶせる固さ Start thin and then gradually increase thickness	歯ぐきで噛める固さ Baby should be able to marsh with the gums
穀類 Cereal (Rice)	つぶしがゆ Smashed Rice porridge or Ground Rice Porridge	全がゆ Rice Porridge	全がゆ→軟飯 Rice Porridge to Soft-cooked Rice	軟飯→ご飯 Soft-cooked Rice to Cooked Rice
卵 Egg	卵黄 Egg Yolks	卵黄→全卵 Egg Yolks to Whole Egg	全卵 Whole Egg	全卵 Whole Egg

4 先天性代謝異常症などの検査
Congenital metabolic disease examination

●個人情報を聴取する Personal data

お子さんのお名前 Name of Child	生年月日 Birth Date: Year, Month, Day
性別 Sex	住所・電話番号 Address・Phone number

●先天性代謝異常症等検査　Congenital metabolic disease examination

1．検査の説明　Explain the examination

■生まれてきた赤ちゃんの中には，先天性代謝異常などの病気をもっていることがあります．
Some of babies are born with congenital illness such as congenital Metabolic Disease.

■「先天性代謝異常等検査」では，生後すぐに血液を調べこれらの病気を見つけます．この検査は「新生児スクリーニング」ともいいます．
This test enables newborn babies to be screened for congenital metabolic disease and is called as "Newborn Screening".

■これらの病気をもつ赤ちゃんには知的障害や発育障害などの症状が現れ，時にはショックや肝障害などで命にかかわることもあります．
Babies with such disease may have intellectual or developmental disorders. Some babies may suffer from life-threatening shock or liver function disorder.

■しかし，早期に専門医の治療を受ければ，障害の発生を防ぐことができます．赤ちゃんにとって，この検査を受けることはとても大切です．ぜひ検査を受けられることをおすすめします．
Early treatment by a specialist prevents suffering from such disorders. Therefore, we encourage every baby to undergo this test.

■検査は，生後4～7日目に赤ちゃんのかかとから採血した血液を用いて行います．
A blood sample from a baby's heel will be collected between the fourth and seventh day after birth.

■現在，検査の対象となっているのは，次の6つの病気です．
Currently the following six diseases are tested.
- フェニルケトン尿症　phenylketonuria (PKU)
- メイプルシロップ尿症　Maple Syrup Urine Disease (MSUD)
- ガラクトース血症　Galactosemia
- 先天性副腎過形成症　Congenital adrenal hyperplasia (CAH)
- ホモシスチン尿症　Homocystinuria
- 先天性甲状腺機能低下症　Congenital hypothyroidism (Cretinism)

■検査料は無料です（産院では，採血のための手数料がかかることがあります）．
This test is usually free of charge. (Occasionally a maternity center may charge for this.)

Part 3　3. 症状を英語で把握する：英語を使った小児科診療・各論

5　よくみる症状
Frequent symptoms

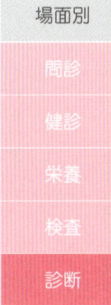

●よくみる症状　Frequent symptoms

1．症状を聞く　Hearing the symptoms

■ どのような症状がありますか
What kind of symptom does he/she has?

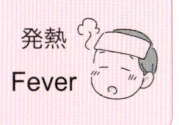

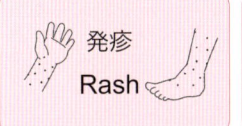

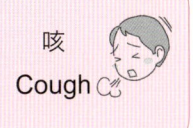

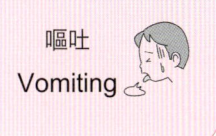

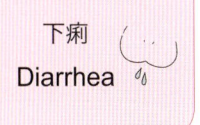

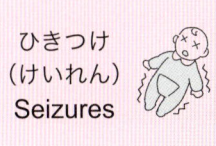

| 発熱 Fever | 発疹 Rash | 咳 Cough | 嘔吐 Vomiting |

| 下痢 Diarrhea | ひきつけ（けいれん） Seizures |

ぐったりしている Extremely weak	寒気 Chills	頭痛 Headache
かゆい Itchy	腫れている Swollen	胃の不調/むかつき Upset stomach
めまいがする Dizziness	胸痛 Chest pain	鼻水が出る Runny nose
吐き気 Nausea	便秘 Constipation	食欲がない No appetite
腹痛 Stomachache	呼吸が早い Fast breathing	のどの痛み Sore throat
泣き止まない Cry nonstop	顔色が悪い Pale	おねしょ Bedwetting

65

■その症状は，いつから始まりましたか？
When did he/she has this symptom?
☐ほんのさきほどから　Very recently
☐１時間まで　One hour ago
☐今朝から　First thing in the morning
☐昨日の夜から　Since last night
☐昨日から　Since yesterday
☐２，３日前から　A couple days ago
☐先週から　Since last week
☐先月から　Since last month
☐昨年から　Since last year

■その症状の頻度はどれくらいですか？
How frequently does he/she has feel this symptom?
☐ときどき　Occasionally
☐しばしば　Often
☐いつも　Most of the time
☐継続してずっと　All the time＝always
☐はじめて　This is the first time
☐以前にあった　He/She has had it before once or twice
☐２回目　This is the second time that he/she has…
☐ほとんど～ない　Almost never＝rarely

2．身体の部位　Part of the body

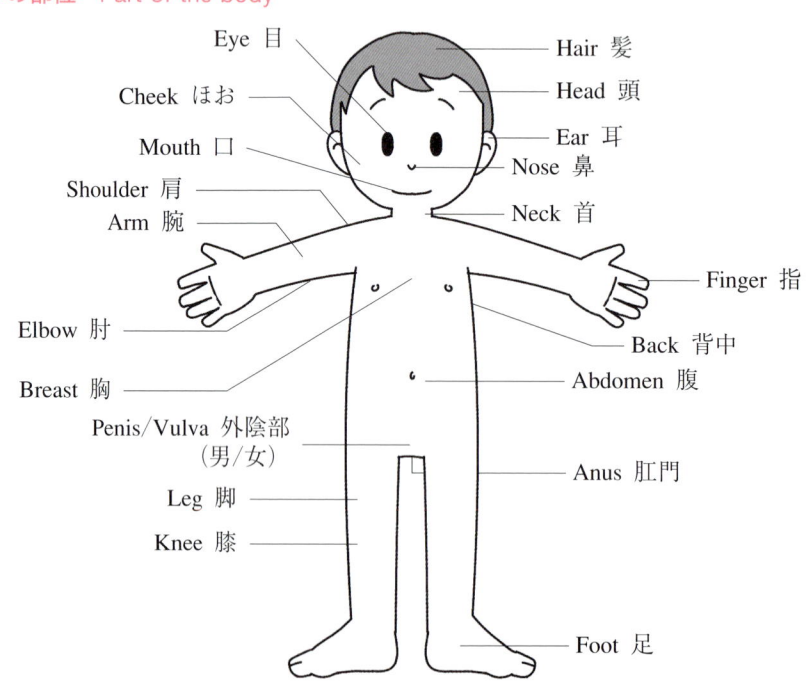

Eye 目
Cheek ほお
Mouth 口
Shoulder 肩
Arm 腕
Elbow 肘
Breast 胸
Penis/Vulva 外陰部
（男/女）
Leg 脚
Knee 膝

Hair 髪
Head 頭
Ear 耳
Nose 鼻
Neck 首
Finger 指
Back 背中
Abdomen 腹
Anus 肛門
Foot 足

4章

病気を英語で説明する
（英語を使った小児科診療・病名編）

To explain the patient's disease

The aim of this chapter

患者に病名を説明するときの会話例．
☝があるところは，症状などを指さしで聞き出し，☑印のところは✓をして説明を一目で理解してもらうのに役立ちます．

Part 4　4. 病名を英語で説明する：英語を使った小児科診療・病名編

1 かぜ症候群
Common cold

●こんな病気　Overview
■かぜ症候群は，鼻やのどのウイルス感染症の総称です．
　The common cold is a general term for viral infection of the nose or throat.
　・Infection　感染症

●原　因　Cause
■かぜ症候群は，たくさんの種類のウイルスによって起こります．
　主なウイルスは，ライノウイルスとコロナウイルスです．
　There are many different viruses that cause a common cold.
　The most common viruses are rhinoviruses and coronaviruses.
■かぜ症候群を起こすウイルスは，咳などを介してうつります．
　Cold viruses can be transmitted in droplets sprayed from the coughs.
　・Rhinoviruses　ライノウイルス
　・Coronaviruses　コロナウイルス

●症　状　Symptoms
■症状は，鼻水，鼻づまり，のどの痛み，咳などです．
　The symptoms of a cold are：
　・Runny nose
　・Nasal congestion
　・Sore throat
　・Cough
■症状は治療なしでも，1 週間以内に良くなります．
　Most colds clear by themselves within a week.
　・Within a week　1 週間以内

●診　断　Diagnosis
■多くの場合，医師の診断が必要になることはありません．
　Most cold do not require a medical diagnosis.
■血液検査や胸部エックス線検査，咽頭検査が行われることもあります．
　Sometimes, they may reguire such tests as bloodtests, chest X rays and throat swab culture test.
　□咽頭培養　Throat swab culture
　□血液検査　Blood test
　□胸部エックス線検査　Chest X-ray

68

1. かぜ症候群　Common cold

●治　療　Treatment

■ 多くの場合，治療が必要となることはありません．
　休養をとったり，水分を補給したりしましょう．
　Most colds clear up by themselves. Children should get plenty of rest and drink liquids.

■ かぜ症候群はウイルス感染症なので，抗菌薬の使用はおすすめできません．
　Antibacterial agent are not prescribed to treat the common cold which is a viral infection.
　・Antibacterial agent　抗菌薬

●合併症　Complications

■ かぜ症候群は，中耳炎や副鼻腔炎を合併することがあります．
　The common cold sometimes has complication such as otitis media and sinusitis.
　・Otitis media　中耳炎
　・Sinusitis　副鼻腔炎

保護者へのアドバイス　Advice to parents

★ 子どもには，アセトアミノフェンという解熱薬を使用します．
Fever reducer named Acetaminophen is used for children.

★ 発熱をしていても，子どもが元気で食欲もあれば，解熱薬を使用する必要はありません．
There is no need to use a fever reducer for children with a fever, but with usual appetite and activity.

★ 熱を下げると，食欲がでたり，眠れたりする場合には，使用します．
しかし，解熱薬は使用しすぎないようにしましょう．
Fever reducer is used if it is expected to recover appetite and/or to improve sleep quality, but do not overuse.

★ 熱があるときは，熱が発散するように薄着にしたりするなど，服装を調節しましょう．
Try to undress to reduce fever.

★ 機嫌が良く，食欲があり，活気があれば，発熱していても，様子をみて良いでしょう．
Try to observe your child if he/she is in a good mood, with good appetite, and in vigor despite fever.

★ ぐったりしている場合，活気がない場合には，再度受診しましょう．
Return to visit the physician if he/she seems to be extremely tired or lacks energy.

病名カテゴリー別

呼吸器
循環器
神経・精神
アレルギー
消化器
泌尿器
外傷
感染症
内分泌・代謝
耳・鼻・咽喉
皮膚

Part 4　4. 病名を英語で説明する：英語を使った小児科診療・病名編

2　インフルエンザ
Influenza

● こんな病気　Overview

■ インフルエンザは，インフルエンザウイルスによって起こる感染症です．流行しやすいのは主に A と B です．

Influenza is an infectious illness caused by influenza virus.
Most influenza outbreaks are caused by influenza Type A or B.

■ インフルエンザの流行は，毎年冬に流行します（主に 10～4 月）．

Seasonal flu is a very common illness that occurs every year, usually during the winter months (October to April in Japan).

■ インフルエンザは，飛沫感染で起こります．

Influenza is spread by infected droplets from coughs or sneezes.

■ 症状がでる 1 日前から，症状が出てからも 5～6 日間は他人を感染させる可能性があります．

People with the influenza remain infectious since 1 day before showing symptoms and for up to 5-6 days after having the symptoms.

● 症　状　Symptom

■ インフルエンザの症状は，突然の高熱，咳，頭痛，関節痛，などです．

Symptoms for seasonal influenza are：
- Sudden high fever
- Cough
- Headache
- Joint or limb pain

■ 感染後 1～4 日で症状がでて，2～3 日間が症状のピークとなります．5～8 日間の経過で軽快します．

Symptoms develop 1 to 4 days after being infected.
Symptoms will usually peak after 2 to 3 days.
Symptoms resolve in 5 to 8 days.

● 診　断　Diagnosis

■ 症状にもとづいて診断しますが，多くは鼻腔のインフルエンザ検査を行います．

The influenza is diagnosed based on the symptoms and by conducting a nasal swab.

● 治　療　Treatment

■ 抗インフルエンザ薬は，症状がでてから 48 時間以内に使用すると効果的です．症状が軽減します．

Antiviral medicines work best if taken within the first 48 hours after the onset of symptoms. They will relieve the symptoms.

2．インフルエンザ　Influenza

●合併症　Complication

■インフルエンザは脳症や肺炎を合併することがあります．
Influenza may be complicated with brain fever and pneumonia.

保護者へのアドバイス　Advice to parents

★安静にして，水分を補給しましょう．
Children should get plenty of rest and drink liquids.

★アスピリンを使用してはいけません．アスピリンはライ症候群との関与が示唆されています．
Child should not take aspirin. Aspirin is associated with a serious illness called Reye Syndrome.

病名カテゴリー別

呼吸器
循環器
神経・精神
アレルギー
消化器
泌尿器
外傷
感染症
内分泌・代謝
耳・鼻・咽喉
皮膚

3 溶連菌感染症
Group A Streptococcal infections (GAS Infections)

Part 4　4. 病名を英語で説明する：英語を使った小児科診療・病名編

●こんな病気　Overview
- 溶連菌感染症とは，溶連菌が人に感染して起こる様々な病気です．
  Hemolytic streptococcus, when transmitted to human, causes a variety of diseases, called Group A streptococcal (GAS) infections.
- 咽頭炎や皮膚感染症，猩紅熱など急性の感染症と，リウマチ熱や糸球体腎炎などのように時間がたって発症する病気もあります．
  Sore throat, skin infections and scarlet fever are acute infections, and rheumatic fever and glomerulonephritis occur after a while.

●原　因　Cause
- 溶連菌は，のどや鼻の分泌物，皮膚病変によって感染します．
  Many GAS infections are spread when a child comes in direct contact with an infected person's skin lesions or secretions from his/her throat or nose.

●症　状　Symptom
- 3歳未満では症状が軽くすみます．しかし，3歳以上の場合には咽頭痛，扁桃に白苔が付着した咽頭の発赤，発熱がみられます．
  When group A streptococcus infects a child younger than 3 years, the symptoms tend to be milder. However a child older than 3 years is infected, he/she may have more serious symptoms such as a high fever, a red and sore throat with white patches of pus on the tonsils.
- 潜伏期間は2～5日です．
  An infected child will become ill 2 to 5 days after being exposed to streptococcal bacteria.

●診　断　Diagnosis
- A群溶連菌迅速診断キット綿棒で，のどの菌を採取し検査します．数分で診断できます．
  Samples from the throat are taken with a cotton-tipped stick from GAS quick testing kit to specify the bacteria within minutes.

●治　療　Treatment
- 溶連菌感染症の治療は，抗菌薬です．ペニシリン系抗菌薬を10～14日間使用します．
  Antibacterial agent are used for treatments. Penicillin is taken orally for 10 to 14 days.

●合併症　Complication
- 溶連菌感染症はリウマチ熱や急性糸球体腎炎に合併することがあります．
  GAS Infections sometimes has complication such as rheumatic fever and acute glomerulonephritis.

3. 溶連菌感染症　Group A Streptococcal infections (GAS Infections)

保護者へのアドバイス　Advice to parents

★症状が消えても，抗菌薬の内服をつづけましょう．
　Don't stop using antibacterial drugs even if the child does not show symptoms anymore.

★抗菌薬を1〜2日内服後，発熱や発疹が治まり元気があれば，登校・登園してもかまいません．
　After taking the antibiotics for 1 or 2 days, if the child recovers his/her energy without fever and rash, he/she can go to preschool or school.

【リウマチ熱　Rheumatism Fever】

★主な症状は，心炎，多発性関節炎，発疹（輪状紅斑），皮下結節，不随意運動です．
　Primary symptoms include carditis (heart problem), multi-articular inflammation, rash (erythema marginatum), subcutaneous nodules, involuntary movements.

★溶連菌感染症から数週間後に発症することがあります．
　Sometimes, this occurs several weeks after hemolytic streptococcal infection.

【急性糸球体腎炎　Acute Glomerulonephritis】

★3大症状（trias）は，血尿，浮腫，高血圧です．
　Three typical symptoms are hematuria, edema and hypertension.

★咽頭炎からは1〜2週間後，皮膚感染からは3〜6週間後に発症することがあります．
　Sometimes, this occurs 1 to 2 weeks after pharyngitis, or 3 to 6 weeks after skin infection.

★治療は，水分および塩分制限，安静にすることです．
　During treatment, hydration, salt restriction and rest are important.

★高血圧が著しい時には，抗圧薬を使います．
　When the pressure soars, hypotensive drugs are used.

★予後は良好です．
　Prognosis is good.

4 肺炎
Pneumonia

●こんな病気　Overview

■肺の感染症を，"肺炎"と呼びます．

The word pneumonia means "infection of the lung."

●原因　Cause

■肺炎の多くは，ウイルスと細菌によって起こる病気です．
ウイルスでは，RS ウイルス，インフルエンザ，パラインフルエンザ，アデノウイルスなど．細菌では，肺炎球菌，インフルエンザ菌，マイコプラズマ，クラミジアなど．

Mostly pneumonia results from an viral and/or bacterial infection.

Such viruses are, respiratory Syncytial Virus (RSV), influenza, parainfluenza, and adenovirus.

Such bacteria are：
- *Streptococcus pneumoniae*
- *Haemophilus influenzae*
- *Mycoplasma pneumoniae*
- *Chlamidophilia pneumoniae*

■肺炎を起こすウイルスや菌は，感染者のつばや粘液などをせきや直接的に接取することで感染します．

Viruses and bacteria are spread through coughing or direct contact with the infected person's saliva or mucus.

●症状　Symptom

■肺炎の症状は，通常，発熱とせきです．

Pneumonia usually produces a fever and a cough.

■呼吸障害を起こすこともあります．症状としては，頻呼吸，努力性呼吸などです．

Sometimes pneumonia causes breathing problems, such as fast breathing rate or labored breathing.

●診断　Diagnosis

■肺炎は，通常症状と身体所見によって診断されますが，胸部エックス線が肺炎の診断に役立ちます．

Usually pneumonia is diagnosed based on the symptoms and the physical findings a chest X-ray can show pneumonia in the lungs.

- □胸部エックス線　Chest X-ray
- □胸部 CT　Chest CT
- □血液検査　Blood test
- □痰培養　Sputum culture

4. 肺 炎 Pneumonia

●治 療　Treatment

■ウイルス性肺炎は対症療法となります．通常は，数日の経過で良くなります．しかし，咳が残る場合があります．
For viral pneumonia, supportive measures are used. It usually improves after a few days, although the cogh may linger for a while.

■細菌性肺炎の場合には，抗菌薬で治療します．
To treat bacterial pneumonia, antibacterial agent are used.

保護者へのアドバイス　Advice to parents

★発熱と咳がつづくと，食欲が低下する場合があります．水分を補給しましょう．
In case of a persistent fever and cough and sometimes loss of appetite, try to give lots of fluids.

★呼吸が苦しそうで，顔色が悪い時は，再度受診しましょう．
Return to the physician, if the child has difficulty breathing and looks pale.

5 急性中耳炎
Acute otitis media

● こんな病気　Overview
■ 中耳炎は，突然起こる中耳の感染症です．
Acute otitis media is a sudden, short-term middle ear infection.

● 原　因　Cause
■ 風邪の場合，膿でいっぱいになります．
While a patient has a cold, the middle ear gets filled with fluid or mucus.

● 症　状　Symptom
■ 中耳炎の症状は，主に発熱と耳の痛みです．
Primary symptoms of acute otitis media are a fever and an earache.
■ 鼓膜がやぶれ，中耳の膿がでてくる場合もあります．
Sometimes pressure on the ear drum breaks through (perforates) the membrane, releasing the fluid.

● 診　断　Diagnosis
■ 中耳炎の診断は，耳鏡による診察により行われます．
Acute otitis media is diagnosed by using an instrument called an auriscope or otoscope.
■ 通常，鼓膜はピンク色ですが，中耳炎の場合には発赤や黄色調になったりします．
The ear drum is usually pink in color but in otitis media it becomes reddish or yellowish.

● 治　療　Treatment
■ 多くの場合，治療なしで良くなります．一般的には抗菌薬が使用されます．
Most of acute otitis media cases clear up without any treatment. In general, antibacterial agent is prescribed.

● 合併症　Complication
☐ 乳様突起炎（乳突洞炎）　Mastoiditis
☐ 髄膜炎　Meningitis

保護者へのアドバイス　Advice to parents

★ 乳児の場合には，特別決まった症状を起こすわけではありません．
It does not cause any specific symptoms to babies.

5．急性中耳炎　Acute otitis media

Column 7

体温，体重，身長を説明する
Body temperature, weight, height

とくに，ふだん，体温をカ氏で測り体重や身長をポンドやフィートで表現している国からきた人には，セ氏やキログラムで説明しても，ピンときません．この換算表を見せながら，使い慣れた単位で説明するととても喜ばれます．

体温(セ氏とカ氏の換算表)

セ氏 Celsius (°C)	カ氏 Fahrenheit (°F)
35	95.0
36	96.8
37	98.6
38	100.4
39	102.0
40	104.0

(°F＝9/5×°C＋32)

体重(キログラムとポンドの換算表)

キログラム (kg)	ポンド (lb)
3	6.61
5	11.0
10	22.1
20	44.1
30	66.1
40	88.2
50	110.2
60	132.3
70	154.3

1 ポンド＝0.4536 キログラム
※ポンドは小数第2位以下を四捨五入した

身長(センチメートルとフィート・インチの換算表)

センチメートル (cm)	フィート・インチ (ft) (in)
50	1'8"
60	1'12"
70	2'4"
80	2'8"
90	2'11"
100	3'3"
110	3'7"
120	3'11"
130	4'3"
140	4'7"
150	4'11"
160	5'3"

1 foot＝30.48 cm, 1 inch＝2.54cm
※インチは小数点以下四捨五入した

6 急性胃腸炎
Gastroenteritis

● こんな病気　Overview

■ 急性胃腸炎は，胃や腸の感染症です．

Gastroenteritis is an infection of the stomach and intestines.

■ 症状が重い場合には，入院が必要となる場合があります．脱水を起こすかも知れないからです．

Sometimes, hospital treatment may be needed when the symptoms get serious, for fear of denydration.

● 原　因　Cause

■ 急性胃腸炎は，ロタウイルスなどのウイルス感染や，多くの細菌感染で起こります．

Gastroenteritis can be caused by viral infections such as the Rotavirus or by a number of different bacteria.

■ 急性胃腸炎は感染しやすい病気です．ですので，衛生状態を良くすることが重要です．

Most forms of gastroenteritis are highly infectious.
Therefore, it is essential to practice good hygiene (wash your hands after using the toilet and before preparing food).

● 症　状　Symptom

■ 主な症状は，下痢と嘔吐です．

Primary symptoms are diarrhea and vomiting.

■ 通常は症状は軽く，数日でよくなります．

The symptoms of gastroenteritis are normally mild and most symptoms will pass within a few days without treatment.

● 診　断　Diagnosis

■ 便検査を行います．特別な細菌がいるかどうか検査をします．

I will stool samples are taken to identify specific bacteria.

■ 血液検査や尿検査が行われる場合もあります．

Sometimes, blood and urine tests may be performed to rule out other conditions.

● 治　療　Treatment

■ 急性胃腸炎の治療は，下痢や嘔吐によって失われた水分を補給することです．

Treatment of gastroenteritis involves replacing the fluids lost from diarrhea and vomiting.

■ 急性胃腸炎に対して，抗菌薬の使用は推奨されていません．

Antibacterial agent are not typically used to treat gastroenteritis.

■ ただし特定の細菌に対しては，抗菌薬が使用される場合もあります．

If a specific bacterial infection is identified, antibacterial agent is prescribed.

6．急性胃腸炎　Gastroenteritis

●合併症　Complication

■急性胃腸炎の主な合併症は，脱水です．
Primary complication of gastroenteritis is dehydration.

■脱水の症状は，脱力感，口のかわき，やつれ顔，目のくぼみなど様々です．
脱水の程度がひどい時には，点滴が必要です．
Symptoms of dehydration include, listlessness, dry mouth, pinched face, sunken eyes.
In more serious cases, hospital treatment to administer intravenous fluids and nutrients will be required.

--- 保護者へのアドバイス　Advice to parents ---

★脂肪や糖分の多い食事は避けましょう．
Avoid fatty foods and foods with high amounts of sugar.

Part 4　4. 病名を英語で説明する：英語を使った小児科診療・病名編

7　食中毒
Food poisoning, Food contamination

●こんな病気　Overview
■食中毒は，細菌やウイルス，寄生虫，毒素，化学物質などに汚染された飲食物を摂食することによって起こる病気です．
Food poisoning is an illness caused by consuming food or drink that has been contaminated by bacteria, viruses, parasites, toxins and chemicals.

●原　因　Cause
1．汚染の原因　Sources of contamination
- □細菌　Bacteria：カンピロバクター，サルモネラ，リステリア，大腸菌，腸炎ビブリオ　Campylobacter, Salmonella, Listeria, Escherichia coli, Vibrio parahaemolyticus
- □ウイルス　Viruses：ロタウイルス，ノロウイルス，腸内アデノウイルス　rotavirus, norovirus, enteric adenorirus
- □寄生虫　Parasites：日本では寄生虫による食中毒の発生はまれです．クリプトスポリジウム，ジルアジア　In Japan, food poisoning from parasites is rare. Cryptosporidium, Giardia
- □毒素　Toxins：油っこい魚　oily fish

●症　状　Symptom
■食中毒の主な症状は，吐き気，嘔吐，下痢です．
Primary symptoms of food poisoning are nausea, vomiting, and diarrhea.
■食中毒の症状は，通常1週間以内で軽快します．
The symptoms of food poisoning will normally pass within a week.

●診　断　Diagnosis
■食中毒の診断は，症状がひどい場合，治療にもかかわらず長引く場合，脱水ある場合，アウトブレイクしている場合に行われます．
Assessing for food poisoning is needed only if symptoms are severe, symptoms persist despite treatment, patients are showing signs of dehydration, and/or there has been an outbreak.
■症状と飲食物の摂食歴をたずねます．
Patients are questioned on their symptoms and any ways they could have come into contact with contaminated food or liquid.
■血液検査，便培養を行うこともあります．
Sometimes samples from blood and/or stool might be tested.

7．食中毒　Food poisoning, Food contamination

●治　療　Treatment
■食中毒の治療は，下痢や嘔吐によって失われた水分を補給することです．
Treatment for food poisoning involves replacing the fluids lost by diarrhea and vomiting.

●予　防　Prevention
■食中毒の一番の予防は，衛生状態の改善です．
The best way to prevent food poisoning is to practice good food hygiene.

保護者へのアドバイス　Advice to parents

★脱水にならないように，水分を補給しましょう．
Try to give lots of fluids to avoid dehydration.

★すぐに吐き出して水分がとれない時，おしっこの量が少ない時，活気がなく顔色が悪い時は，再度受診しましょう．
Return to the physician, if you see the child vomits and doesn't drink water, urinates little, loses energy or looks pale.

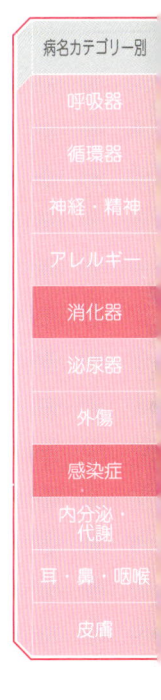

8 尿路感染症
Urinary Tract Infection (UTI)

●こんな病気　Overview

■尿路感染症は尿路に起きた感染症です．
尿路とは腎臓，尿管，膀胱，尿道までのことです．
Urinary tract infection (UTI) is an infection of any part of the urinary system.
The urinary system is made up of the kidneys, the ureters, the bladder and the urethra.

■感染が起きた部分により，上部尿路感染症(腎盂腎炎)，下部尿路感染症(膀胱炎，尿道炎)に分かれます．
There are two different types of UTI：
Upper UTI：pyelonephritis
Lower UTI：cystitis, urethritis

■上部尿路感染症は，下部尿路感染症よりも重症です．なぜなら腎臓へのダメージを起こす可能性があるからです．
Upper UTI is potentially more serious than lower UTI, because there is a possibility of kidney damage.

●原　因　Cause

■尿路感染症は細菌が尿道から入ってきて，感染を起こすことがほとんどです．その細菌の多くは大腸菌です．
Mostly urinary tract infection (UTI) is caused when bacteria, typically Escherichia. Coli, enter and infect the urinary tract.

●症　状　Symptom

■3歳未満のお子さんでは，尿路感染症に特徴的な症状が乏しいことがあります．
UTI in children, particularly those under 3 years old, can be difficult to identify.

■尿路感染症の症状は，頻尿，排尿時痛，血尿，発熱，腹痛などです．
Symptoms include：
・Increased urination
・Pain while urinating
・Blood in the urine
・Fever
・Abdominal pain

●診　断　Diagnosis

■尿路感染症は尿検査と尿培養で診断されます．尿培養は適切な抗菌薬を選ぶのに必要です．
UTI is diagnosed by urine analysis and urine culture. A urine culture sample is required in order to prescribe the most appropriate antibacterial agent to treat it.

8．尿路感染症　Urinary Tract Infection(UTI)

☐尿検査　Urine analysis
☐尿培養　Urine culture
☐血液検査　Blood test
☐超音波検査　Ultrasound scan, Sonography
☐排尿時膀胱造影　VCG（Voiding cystography）

●治　療　Treatment

■上部尿路感染症は，次の観点から早く治療をすることが大事です．感染症を治癒するためと，腎臓の損傷を減らすためです．
It is important to treat upper UTI immediately to cure the infection and to reduce kidney damage.

■尿路感染症は，抗菌薬で治療します．上部尿路感染症の場合，2週間程度の治療が必要です．
Antibacterial agent are prescribed to treat UTI. For upper UTI, about 2 week-treatment is necessary.

●予　後　Prognosis

■反復性の尿路感染症は膀胱炎，膀胱尿管逆流を起こすことがあります．
Sometimes recurrent UTI causes cystitis and/or vesicoureteral reflux.

保護者へのアドバイス　Advice to parents

★尿路感染症を予防するためのアドバイスは，次の通りです．
前から後ろへおしりを拭く，陰部を清潔に保つ，定期的に排尿する，です．
UTI can be prevented by：
・Wiping from front to back.
・Cleaning the foreskin of the penis or vulvae.
・Urinating frequently.

9 突発性発疹
Exanthema subitum, Roseola infantum

●こんな病気　Overview

■突然の高熱をもって発症し，解熱と同時に発疹が出現する急性ウイルス性疾患です．
Exanthema subitum is an acute viral disease with sudden high fever and is characterized by a rash appearance as temperature drops rapidly to normal.

■突発性発疹は，生後6か月～2歳頃までに起こる病気です．
6か月～1歳頃の乳児によくみられ，生まれて初めての発熱であることが多いです．
Exanthema subitum most often occurs in 6 to 24 months old children.
Many babies experience such a high fever for the first time.

●原　因　Cause

■原因は，ウイルス〔おもにヒトヘルペスウイルス6（HHV-6）およびヒトヘルペスウイルス7（HHV-7）〕です．
Exanthema subitum is a viral infection caused primary by human herpesvirus 6 (HHV-6) human herpesvirus 7 (HHV-7).

●症　状　Symptom（図）

■3～7日間の高熱が続きます．その後，解熱とともに発疹が全身に出ます．
発疹は数時間から数日続く場合もあります．
Children will typically have a high fever for 3 to 7 days.
After their temperature drops, they will have a rash all over the body.
The rash could last several days.

●診　断　Dignosis

■症状と経過で診断します．
Exanthema subitum is diagnosed from the symptoms and the course.

●治　療　Treatment

■突発性発疹の治療はありません．
There is no specific treatment for Exanthema Subitum.

●合併症　Complication

■熱の高い時に，けいれんを起こすことがあります．
Some children have seizures associated with high fever.

9．突発性発疹　Exanthema subitum, Roseola infantum

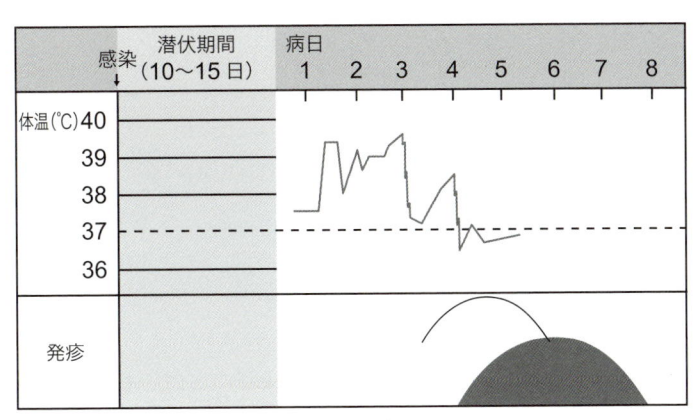

図　経過例

保護者へのアドバイス　Advice to parents

★熱が下がるまで，他の子どもとあそばせないようにしましょう．
Don't let your child play with other children until the fever subsides.

★熱が下がってからは，たとえ発疹があっても通常の生活に戻してかまいません．
After the fever has gone, your child can return to childcare or preschool and resume normal contact with other children even if a rash has appeared.

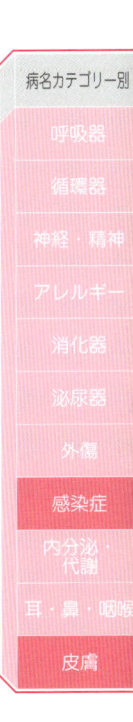

Part 4　4. 病名を英語で説明する：英語を使った小児科診療・病名編

10　熱性けいれん
Febrile seizures

●こんな病気　Overview

■熱性けいれんは，発熱に伴って起こるけいれんです．
　Febrile seizures are triggered by fever.

■熱性けいれんは，脳炎や髄膜炎などの中枢神経感染症などけいれんの原因になるような異常をみとめないものです．
　Febrile seizures may not be symptoms of central nervous system problems such as encephalitis and meningitis.

■6か月から5歳くらいまでの小児100人のうち3〜4人に起こりますが，主に1〜2歳です．
　Febrile seizures occur in 3-4 of every 100 children 6 months-5 years old. The age group most affected is 12-24 month old children.

・Encephalitis　脳炎
・Meningitis　髄膜炎

●原　因　Cause

■熱性けいれんの原因は，はっきりしないことが多いです．
　In many cases, the cause of febrile seizures is unknown.

●特　徴　Characteristic

■熱性けいれんは，熱があがって数時間に起こることが多いです．
　Febrile seizures mostly occur during the first few hours of a fever.

■熱性けいれんが止まった後，子どもの意識は元にもどります．
　けいれんは通常1分未満のことが多いですが，15分間続くこともあります．
　After a febrile seizure the child can quickly return to normal.
　Seizures usually last less than 1 minute but, rarely they can last for up to 15 minutes.

●検　査　Test

■熱の原因を調べます．髄膜炎のような重症な感染症の有無を評価するために腰椎穿刺を行うこともあります．
　Causes of the fever are examined. A spinal tap may be done to be sure the child does not have a serious infection like meningitis.

　□血液検査　Blood test
　□腰椎穿刺　Spinal tap
　□髄液検査　Test for cerebrospinal fluid
　□頭部CT　Pictures of the brain using computed tomography (CT scan)
　□MRI　Magnetic resonance imaging (MRI)
　□脳波　Electroencephalogram (EEG)

10. 熱性けいれん　Febrile seizures

● 治　療　Treatment

一般的に，一回の単純型熱性けいれんに対して，抗けいれん薬の予防的な使用は勧められていません．けいれんが長い時間であった場合や，けいれんを繰り返す場合には，抗けいれん薬の予防投与を考えても良いかもしれません．

Generally for a one-time seizure or simple febrile seizures, preventive medication such as anticonvulsant drugs are not recommended.

If seizures are prolonged or repeated, preventive medication may be necessary.

● 予　後　Prognosis

熱性けいれんの予後は良好です．

Febrile seizures do not cause long-term health problems.

保護者へのアドバイス　Advice to parents

★熱さましは熱を下げることはできますが，熱性けいれんの予防にはなりません．
Feber reducers can help lower a fever, but they do not prevent febrile seizures.

★子どもがけいれんを起こしたら，吐物を詰まらせないようにしましょう．
If your child is having a seizure, roll your child to his/her side to prevent choking in case of vomiting.

★けいれんが起きても，舌をかみきることはありません．
During a seizure, there is no risk of your child swallowing his/her tongue.

★けいれんが2～3分以内におさまらない場合には，救急車を呼びましょう．
If seizures do not stop within 2-3 minutes, call 119 for an ambulance.

11 手足口病
Hand-foot-and mouth disease

● こんな病気　Overview

- 発熱と発疹をひき起こすウイルス感染症です．
  This is a viral infection, which causes fever and eruptions.
- 発疹が手・足・口にできるため，ユニークな名前がついています．
  Since eruptions appear on the hands, foot, and mouth, it has a funny name.
- 多くは夏に流行し，「夏かぜ」の1つとなっています．
  Most cases outbreak during summer. It is one of the "summertime colds".
  - Viral infection　ウイルス感染症

● 原　因　Cause

- ヘルパンギーナと同様にエンテロウイルスが原因で，のどや鼻から感染します．
  The same as herpangina, enterovirus is the cause, infected through throat or nose.
- エンテロウイルスの中には多くの種類があるため，2〜3回かかることもあります．
  Since there are many different kinds in enterovirus, patient might be infected multiple times.
  - Enterovirus　エンテロウイルス

● 症　状　Symptom

- 感染してから3〜4日後に，発熱，手・足・口の中・おしりなどに発疹が出現します．
  3 to 4 days after infected, fever and eruptions develop on the hands, foot, in the mouth, and buttocks.
- 約1週間で治りますが，まれに髄膜炎などの合併症を起こすことがあります．
  It goes away in about 1 week. Rarely complications such as meningitis occur.
  - Meningitis　髄膜炎

● 検　査　Test

- 多くは症状から診断しますが，血液・のど・便検査などでウイルスを特定することもあります．
  In most cases, diagnosis is based on the symptoms. Samples from blood, throat, and stool might be tested to specify the virus.
  - ☐ 血液検査　Blood test
  - ☐ のどの検査　Throat test
  - ☐ 便検査　Stool test

11. 手足口病　Hand-foot-and mouth disease

●治　療　Treatment

■特別な治療法はありません．発熱や口の痛みなどの症状を和らげる治療を行います．

There is no specific treatment for this disease. Treatment to relieve the symptoms such as fever and pain in the mouth is given.

保護者へのアドバイス　Advice to parents

★口の痛みで飲食ができない場合は，プリンやアイスクリームなどのやわらかく冷たい食べ物や水分を少しずつ与えます．

When pain in the mouth prevents your children from taking food and drinks, give them something soft and cold such as custard pudding or ice cream or fluid small amount at a time.

★手足口病にかかると，ウイルスは長期間便に排泄されることがあります．ですので，普段から手洗いやうがいを心がけるとよいでしょう．

When you get Hand-foot-and-mouth disease, virus may be excreted with bowel movement for a long time. Washing hands and gargle often as daily routine are recommended.

★熱もなく元気があれば，日常生活や登園・登校に制限はありません．

If you do not have fever and feel fine, there is no restriction with daily activities and attending school.

12 ヘルパンギーナ
Herpangina

Part 4　4. 病名を英語で説明する：英語を使った小児科診療・病名編

●こんな病気　Overview

■発熱とのどの痛みをひき起こすウイルス感染症です．
　This is viral infection, which causes fever and sore throat.

■「ヘルパンギーナ」の言葉の由来は，ドイツ語の「ヘルプ＝ヘルペス（水ぶくれ）」「アンギーナ＝のどの炎症（赤くはれて痛いこと）」と言われています．
　Origin of "herpangina" is from German words : "herpes (vesicular eruption)" and "angina (quinsy)."

■多くは夏に流行し，「夏かぜ」の1つとなっています．
　Most cases outbreak in summer. It is one of the "summertime colds."

・Viral infection　ウイルス感染症

●原　因　Cause

■手足口病と同様にエンテロウイルスが原因で，のどや鼻から感染します．
　The same as hand-foot and mouth disease, enterovirus is the cause and infected through throat or nose.

■エンテロウイルスの中には多くの種類があるため，2～3回かかることもあります．
　Since there are many different kinds in enterovirus, patient might be infected multiple times.

・Enterovirus　エンテロウイルス

●症　状　Symptom

■感染してから3～4日後に，発熱とのどの痛みが出現します．
　3 to 4 days after infected, fever and sore throat develop.

■のどの奥には小さな水ぶくれがみられ，その痛みのため飲食ができなくなることがあります．
　Small blisters in the back of the throat appear. This may be too painful to eat and drink.

■1週間程度で治りますが，まれに髄膜炎などの合併症を起こすことがあります．
　It goes away in about 1 week. Rarely complications such as meningitis occur.

・Complication　合併症
・Meningitis　髄膜炎

●検　査　Test

■多くは症状から診断しますが，血液・のど・便検査などでウイルスを特定することもあります．
　In most cases, diagnosis is based on the symptoms. Samples from blood, throat, and stool might be tested to specify the virus.

□血液検査　Blood test

12. ヘルパンギーナ　Herpangina

　　□のどの検査　Throat test
　　□便検査　Stool test

● 治　療　Treatment
■特別な治療法はありません．発熱や口の痛みなどの症状を和らげる治療を行います．
There is no specific treatment for this disease. Treatment to relieve the symptoms such as fever and soreness in the mouth is given.

保護者へのアドバイス　Advice to parents

★口の痛みで飲食ができない場合は，プリンやアイスクリームなどのやわらかく冷たい食べ物や水分を少しずつ与えます．
When soreness in the mouth prevents your children from taking food and drinks, give them something soft and cold such as custard pudding or ice cream or fluid small amount at a time.

★予防するワクチンはないため，普段から手洗いやうがいを心がけるとよいでしょう．
There is no vaccination available to prevent this. Wash hands and gargle frequently and thoroughly daily.

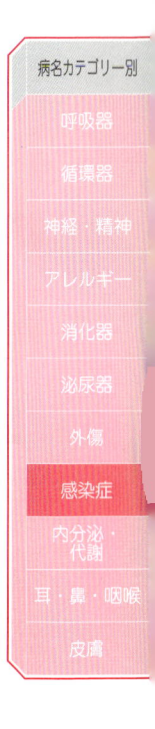

Part 4 4. 病名を英語で説明する：英語を使った小児科診療・病名編

13 麻　疹（はしか）
Measles

●こんな病気　Overview
■高熱と発疹をひき起こす伝染力の強いウイルス感染症です．
This is a highly contagious viral infection which causes high fever and rash.

■多くの国ではワクチン普及によりめずらしい病気となっています．しかし，日本では時に大流行することがあります．
Since vaccination coverage is widely available in most countries, it has become a rare disease.
However, there are times measles epidemics occur in Japan.

・Viral infection　ウイルス感染症

●原　因　Cause
■麻疹ウイルスが原因で，のどや鼻から感染します．
Measles virus is the cause, infection occurs through throat and nose.

■麻疹の患者さんと同じ部屋にいるだけで感染します．
It is so contagious that infected person can transmit it to the others in the same room who are not immune.

・Measles virus　麻疹ウイルス

●症　状　Symptom
■感染して約 10 日後から発熱やせきで始まり，さらに 3～4 日後に体に発疹が出現し，1 週間ほどでしみとなり次第に消えていきます．
About 10 days after infected, it begins with fever and cough. 3 to 4 days after symptoms begin rash spreads on the body, it becomes darker spots, and fades away in 1week.

■時々中耳炎や肺炎，まれに脳炎などの重い合併症が起こることがあります．
Sometimes, complications such as otitis media, pneumonia, and rarely in serious cases, encephalitis may occur.

●検　査　Test
■症状に加え，血液・尿・のどの検査などでウイルスを特定します．
Besides symptoms, samples from blood, urine, and throat are tested to specify the virus.

☐血液検査　Blood test
☐のど検査　Throat test
☐便検査　Stool test

●治　療　Treatment
■特別な治療法はありません．
There is no specific treatment for this disease.

13. 麻 疹（はしか） Measles

- 発熱やせきなどの症状を和らげる治療を行います．
  Treatment to relieve symptoms such as fever and cough is given.
- 中耳炎や肺炎に対しては抗菌薬などを使用することもあります．
  In case complications develop such as otitis media and pneumonia, antibacterial agent may be prescribed.

● 予 防　Prevention

- 有効なワクチンがあります．
  Vaccine is effective.
- 多くの国では麻疹・おたふくかぜ・風疹の混ざったMMRワクチンを2回接種しますが，日本では麻疹・風疹の混ざったMRワクチンを，一般的に1歳，5歳で2回接種します．
  In many countries, MMR vaccine：measles-mumps-rubella immunization is given twice. In Japan, MR vaccine：measles-rubella immunization is given twice at 1 year and 5 years of age.
- 麻疹の患者さんと接触した場合，3日以内であればワクチンを，6日以内であれば免疫グロブリン（血液製剤）を注射すると，麻疹にかからなかったり軽くすんだりすることがあります．
  When exposure to an infected person occurs, if it is within 3 days of the exposure, vaccination is injected. If it is within 6 days of the exposure, immune globulin is injected. By giving injections, measles can be prevented or the symptoms can be mild.

● 薬の副作用　Side effect of medications

- ワクチンを接種した後に，発熱（20〜30％），発疹（10％），注射した部分の赤み（数％）などが出現することがあります．
  Measles vaccine may cause fever（in 20 to 30% of children getting the vaccine）, rash（in 10% of them）, and redness on the injected area（in a few % of them）.

保護者へのアドバイス　Advice to parents

★解熱した後3日までは，幼稚園や学校を休ませる必要があります．
  Until 3 days after fever is lowered, keep your children out of kindergarten or school.

★地球上から麻疹をなくすためには，みんながワクチンを接種することが大切です．
  To eliminate measles, it is important that everyone receives immunization.

14 風疹
Rubella

● こんな病気　Overview

■ 発熱と発疹をひき起こすウイルス感染症です．
This is a viral infection causes fever and rash.

■ 「3日はしか」とも呼ばれ，伝染力も症状もはしか（麻疹）より軽い病気です．
It is called "3-day measles" and compared to measles, it is less contagious with milder symptoms.

・Viral infection　ウイルス感染症

● 原　因　Cause

■ 風疹ウイルスが原因で，のどや鼻から感染します．
Rubella virus is the cause, infection occurs through the throat and nose.

・Rubella virus　風疹ウイルス

● 症　状　Symptom

■ 感染してから2〜3週間後に発熱と麻疹によく似た発疹が出現し，3日前後で消えていきます．
2 to 3 weeks after infected, fever and rash similar to the one with measles appear and fade in around 3 days.

■ 首のリンパ節がはれ，痛みを伴います．
Painful swelling in the lymph nodes on the neck

■ 麻疹ほどの重い合併症は少ないですが，妊娠初期の妊婦さんが風疹ウイルスに感染すると，生まれた赤ちゃんに目の病気・心臓病・難聴などを伴う先天性風疹症候群をひき起こすことがあるため注意が必要です．
There are less severe complications compared to measles, however, pregnant women should take extra precaution. If a mother is infected during early pregnancy, it can cause congenital rubella syndrome such as eye and heart diseases, hearing loss to the unborn baby.

・Congenital rubella syndrome　先天性風疹症候群

● 検　査　Test

■ 症状に加え，血液検査などでウイルスを特定します．
Besides symptoms, blood test is used to specify the virus.

● 治　療　Treatment

■ 特別な治療法はありません．
There is no specific treatment for this disease.

14. 風　疹　Rubella

■発熱などの症状を和らげる治療を行います．
Treatment to reduce fever is given.

●予　防　Prevention

■有効なワクチンがあります．
Vaccine is effective.

■多くの国では麻疹・おたふくかぜ・風疹の混ざったMMRワクチンを2回接種しますが，日本では麻疹・風疹の混ざったMRワクチンを，一般的に1歳，5歳で2回接種します．
In many countries, MMR vaccine：measles-mumps-rubella vaccination is given twice. In Japan, MR vaccine：measles-rubella vaccination is given twice at 1 year and 5 years of age.

●薬の副作用　Side effect of medications

■ワクチンを接種した後に，発熱（20〜30％），発疹（10％），注射した部分の赤み（数％）などが出現することがあります．
Rubella vaccine may cause fever（in 20 to 30% of children getting the vaccine）, rash（in 10% of them）, and redness on the injected area（in a few % of them）.

保護者へのアドバイス　Advice to parents

★発疹が消えるまでは，幼稚園や学校を休ませる必要があります．
Until rash disappears, keep your children out of kindergarten or school.

★先天性風疹症候群を起こさないために，女の子だけでなくみんながワクチンを接種して病気をなくすことが大切です．
To prevent congenital rubella syndrome, it is important that not only girls get vaccination but everybody receives it.

Part 4

4. 病名を英語で説明する：英語を使った小児科診療・病名編

15 おたふくかぜ
Mumps, "Otafuku-cold", Epidemic parotitis

●こんな病気　Overview

■発熱と耳下腺（耳の下の唾液腺）のはれをひき起こすウイルス感染症です．
It is a viral infection which causes fever and swelling of parotid glands (salivary glands under ears).

■「おたふくかぜ」の言葉の由来は，「おたふく」という日本の伝統的なお面のようにほっぺたがはれることから来ています．
The origin of "Otafuku-cold" comes from a Japanese traditional mask 'Otafuku' with round and chubby cheeks since its major symptom is swelling of the cheeks.

■その他「流行性耳下腺炎」，「ムンプス」とも呼ばれています．
Other names are epidemic parotitis and mumps.

■多くの国ではワクチン普及のため発生の少ない病気です．しかし，日本ではワクチン接種が不十分なためしばしば流行します．
Since vaccination coverage is widely available in many countries, it has become a rare disease. In Japan, however, vaccination is not widely applied and epidemics occur sometimes.

- Epidemic parotitis　流行性耳下腺炎
- Mumps　ムンプス

●原　因　Cause

■ムンプスウイルスが原因で，のどや鼻から感染します．
Mumps virus is the cause and infection occurs through the throat and nose.

- Mumps virus　ムンプスウイルス

●症　状　Symptom

■感染してから2〜3週間後に発熱と痛みのある耳下腺のはれが出現します．
2 to 3 weeks after infected, fever and painful swelling of parotid glands develop.

■両方または片方の耳下腺がはれ，約1週間で消えていきます．
Both or one side parotid glands get swollen and disappear about in 1 week.

■ムンプスウイルスは耳下腺のほかに脳・耳・精巣・卵巣も好みますので，ときどき髄膜炎・難聴・精巣炎・卵巣炎などの合併症をひき起こすため注意が必要です．
Precaution may be needed since besides parotid glands, mumps virus may stay in the brain, ears, testicles, and ovaries. Complications such as meningitis, hearing loss, orchitis, and oophoritis may occur.

●検　査　Test

■症状で診断します．
Diagnosis is based on the symptoms.

15. おたふくかぜ　Mumps, "Otafuku-cold", Epidemic parotitis

■血液やだ液の検査などでウイルスを特定することもあります.
Samples from blood or saliva test may be tested to specify the virus.
　☐血液検査　Blood test
　☐だ液検査　Saliva test

●治　療　Treatment
■特別な治療法はありません.
There is no specific treatment for this disease.
■発熱や痛みなどの症状を和らげる治療を行います.
Treatment to relive fever and pain is given.

●予　防　Prevention
■有効なワクチンがあります.
Vaccine is effective.
■多くの国では麻疹・おたふくかぜ・風疹の混ざったMMRワクチンを無料で接種(定期接種)できますが,以前日本ではMMRワクチンによる副作用が多かったため,今でもおたふくかぜ単独のワクチンを個人の判断かつ自己負担で接種(任意接種)することになります.
Though in many countries, MMR vaccine：measles-mumps-rubella vaccination is given at no cost (routine vaccination), in Japan, a single mumps vaccination is still optional and at owns cost. This is because MMR vaccination caused many side effects before.

●薬の副作用　Side effect of medications
■ワクチンを接種した後に,発熱,発疹,注射した部分の赤みなど,またまれに髄膜炎を起こすこともあります.
After receiving vaccination, fever, rash, and redness on the injected area may develop. Rarely this may cause meningitis.
・Meningitis　髄膜炎

保護者へのアドバイス　Advice to parents

★食べ物をかむとアゴに強い痛みがあるため,プリンやゼリー,おかゆなどやわらかい食べ物や飲み物がよいでしょう.
Chewing food causes intense pain to the jaws. Soft food such as custard pudding, jelly, or porridge might be good for your children.

★耳下腺のはれが消えるまで,幼稚園や学校を休ませる必要があります.
Until swelling of parotid glands disappears, keep your children out of kindergarten or school.

★ワクチンの副作用よりおたふくかぜの合併症の方が重いことが多いため,ワクチン接種をおすすめします.
Since complications from mumps are much severe than the one from vaccination, vaccination is recommended.

Part 4　4. 病名を英語で説明する：英語を使った小児科診療・病名編

16　水ぼうそう
Varicella, Chickenpox

● こんな病気　Overview

■ 高熱と水疱（小さな水ぶくれ）をひき起こす伝染力の強いウイルス感染症です．
Ii is a highly contagious viral infection that causes high fever and vesicles (small fluid-filled blisters).

■ 「水痘」とも呼ばれています．
It is also called as "chickenpox", SUITOH in Japanese.

■ 一度かかると，水ぼうそうのウイルスが体内に潜伏し，体力が落ちた時に再び皮膚に出現し，顔や体の一部に水疱ができる「帯状疱疹」をひき起こすことがあります．
Once infected with this, varicella-zoster virus remains dormant in the body. When physical strength declines, the virus re-emerges and causes "shingles," which vesicles develop on the face and body.

■ 多くの国ではワクチン普及のため発生の少ない病気ですが，わが国ではワクチン接種が不十分なためしばしば流行します．
Since vaccination coverage is widely available in many countries, it has become a rare disease. In Japan, however, vaccination is not sufficient and endemic occur sometimes.

・Chickenpox　水痘
・Shingles　帯状疱疹

● 原　因　Cause

■ 水痘／帯状疱疹ウイルスが原因で，のどや鼻から感染します．
Varicella-zoster virus, a member of the herpesvirus family, is the cause. Infection occurs through the throat and nose.

■ 水ぼうそうの患者さんと同じ部屋にいるだけで感染します．
It is so contagious that an infected person can transmit it to others who are in the same room.

● 症　状　Symptom

■ 感染してから2～3週間後に発熱とかゆみのある発疹が体中に次々と出現します．
2 to 3 weeks after infection, fever and itching eruptions develop one after another.

■ 発疹は，小さな赤み・水ぶくれ・かさぶたへと変化し，約1週間で治っていきます．
Eruptions are small red spots and turn to blisters, then become crusts. In about 1 week they fade away.

■ 妊娠中や出産前後に妊婦さんが水ぼうそうにかかると，生まれた赤ちゃんに重い症状や合併症をひき起こすことがあるので注意が必要です．
Pregnant women need extra precaution. If a mother gets infected during pregnancy and before and after the delivery, the baby would get severe symptoms or complications.

16. 水ぼうそう　Varicella, Chickenpox

●検　査　Test
■症状で診断しますが，血液や水疱の検査などでウイルスを特定することもあります．
Diagnosis is based on the symptoms. Samples from blood and vesicle might be used to specify the virus.

●治　療　Treatment
■必要に応じてウイルスを退治する薬を4〜5日間内服します．
Oral antiviral medication is taken for 4 to 5 days if necessary.
■水疱にはかゆみ止めなどの塗り薬を使用します．
For vesicles, topical ointment is used to relieve itching.
■水疱が化膿した場合は抗菌薬を内服します．
If vesicles get infected, oral antibacterial agent is taken.

●予　防　Prevention
■有効なワクチンがあります．
Vaccine is effective.
■多くの国では水ぼうそうのワクチンを無料で接種（定期接種）できますが，日本では個人の判断かつ自己負担で接種（任意接種）することになります．
Though in many countries, varicella vaccine is given at no cost, (routine immunization) in Japan, is still optional and at owns cost.
■水ぼうそうの患者さんと接触した場合，3日以内であればワクチンを注射すると，水ぼうそうにかからなかったり軽くすんだりすることがあります．
When exposure to an infected person occurs, if it is within three days of the exposure, vaccination is injected, varicella can be prevented or the symptoms can be mild.

●薬の副作用　Side effect of medications
■ワクチンを接種した後に，発熱，発疹，注射した部分の赤みなどが起こることがあります．
After receiving vaccination, fever, rash, and redness on the injected area may develop.

保護者へのアドバイス　Advice to parents

★すべての発疹がかさぶたになるまで，幼稚園や学校を休ませる必要があります．
Until all the blisters get crusted, keep your children out of kindergarten or school.

★ウイルス感染症の中では治療薬のある数少ない病気です．
Mediation is available for treating varicella. It is rare that specific medications are available for a viral infectious disease.

17 百日咳
Pertussis, Whooping cough

Part 4　4. 病名を英語で説明する：英語を使った小児科診療・病名編

●こんな病気　Overview

■特徴的な咳発作をひき起こす細菌感染症です．
　This is a bacterial infection which causes characteristic episodes of coughing.

■「Pertussis」はラテン語で「ひどい咳」を意味します．百日近く咳が続くこともあります．
　"Pertussis" means 'severe coughing' in Latin.
　Coughing might last for nearly 100 days.

■最近は大人の間でも流行しており，予防接種をしていない赤ちゃんにうつしてしまうため問題となっています．
　Recently it has become a problem where it outbreaks among adults and spread to babies who are not immune.

●原　因　Cause

■百日咳菌が原因です．のどや鼻から感染します．
　Bordetella pertussis, which is a kind of bacteria, is the cause. Infection occurs through the throat and nose.

　・Bordetella pertussis　百日咳菌

●症　状　Symptom

■感染してから約1週間後にかぜ症状が出現し，さらに1〜2週間後には咳が「コンコンコンコン」と長く続き「ヒューッ」と吸い込む発作をくり返すようになります．
　Common cold symptoms develop about 1 week after infected and in 1 to 2 weeks long hacking coughs start followed by episodes of whooping noise.

■その発作が2〜3週間続き，2〜3か月で咳がなくなります．
　The episodes last for 2 to 3 weeks. Coughing stops in 2 to 3 months.

■乳児は，咳発作ではなく一時的に息が止まり顔が真っ青になることがあります．
　In infants, instead of having episode of coughing, their breathing may temporarily stop and look very pale.

●検　査　Test

■症状，血液や鼻の検査などで診断します．
　Diagnosis is made by symptoms and samples from blood and nose.
　□血液検査　Blood test
　□鼻の検査　Nose test

●治　療　Treatment

■抗菌薬を内服します．
　Antibacterial agent is taken.

17. 百日咳　Pertussis, Whooping cough

●予　防　Prevention

■有効なワクチンがあります．
Vaccine is effective.

■ジフテリア・百日咳・破傷風の混ざったDPT三種混合ワクチンを乳児期に接種します．
DPT vaccine：diphtheria-pertussis-tetanus vaccine is given to infants.

■多くの国ではDPT三種混合ワクチンの接種をさらに追加して予防効果を高めます．しかし，日本での追加の接種は百日咳を含まないDT二種混合ワクチンの接種であるため，大人の百日咳が増えているといわれています．
In many countries DPT boosters are scheduled at childhood immunization. In Japan, however, the booster shots are DT vaccination and pertussis is not included. This may cause the outbreak of pertussis among adults.

●薬の副作用　Side effect of medications

■ワクチンを接種した後に，発熱，発疹，注射した部分の赤み・はれなどが起こることがあります．
After receiving vaccination, fever, rash, and redness on the injected area may develop.

保護者へのアドバイス　Advice to parents

★特徴的な咳発作が消えるまで，幼稚園や学校を休ませる必要があります．
Until episodes of characteristic coughing stop, keep your children out of kindergarten or school.

★咳がひどい時は，部屋の温度や湿度を高めに設定し，水分を十分摂取するとよいでしょう．
If coughing is severe, keep the room temperature and humidity high and give sufficient fluid.

Part 4　4. 病名を英語で説明する：英語を使った小児科診療・病名編

18　川崎病
Kawasaki disease

●こんな病気　Overview

■全身の血管に炎症（赤くはれること）を起こします．
発熱や様々な症状がみられる病気です．

It causes inflammation of blood vessels in the whole body.
There are various symptoms, including fever.

■まれに心臓にダメージを起こすこともあります．

It rarely may damage the heart.
1960年代に川崎富作さん（小児科医）が発見しました．

In 1960s, Dr. Tomisaku Kawasaki (pediatrician) discovered this disease.

・Inflammation of blood vessels　血管の炎症

●原　因　Cause

■原因不明で，主に4歳以下の子どもにみられます．

The cause has not been identified and most of the patients are younger than age 4.

●症　状　Symptom

■以下の6つの症状のうち，5つ以上がみられると川崎病と診断します．

When more than 5 symptoms are observed out of the followed 6 symptoms, it is diagnosed Kawasaki disease.

①高熱が5日以上続きます

1) High fever last for more than 5 days.

②目が赤くなります

2) Eyes get red.

③唇や舌が赤くなります

3) Lips get bright red and tongue gets strawberry color.

④体に赤い発しんが出ます

4) Red skin rashes develop on the body.

⑤手足の先が赤くはれます

5) Swelling of tips of the hand and feet.

⑥首のリンパ節がはれます

6) Lymph nodes in the neck area get swollen.

■心臓へ血液を送る血管（冠動脈）が赤くはれ，コブができることがあります．

Inflammation occurs in the arteries which send blood to the heart (coronary arteries) and this may cause aneurysms.

■コブの中では血液の塊ができやすく，それが血管につまると心臓にダメージを起こします．

In aneurysms, blood clot tends to form and if it gets stuck in the vessels, it damages the heart.

18. 川崎病　Kawasaki disease

- Coronary arteries　冠動脈
- Aneurysms　コブ

● 検　査　Test

■ 血液や尿の検査，胸部エックス線，心電図，心臓超音波検査などを行います．

Blood and urine tests, chest x-ray, ECG, and echocardiogram may be performed.
- ☐ 尿検査　Urine test
- ☐ 胸部エックス線　Chest X-ray
- ☐ 心電図　ECG
- ☐ 心臓超音波検査　Echocardiogram

● 治　療　Treatment

■ 入院し，免疫グロブリン（血液製剤）の点滴やアスピリン（炎症を抑える，血を固まりにくくする）の内服を行います．

Patients are admitted to hospitals and treated with intravenous immunogloblin (blood derivatives) and oral aspirin (anti-inflammatory and anticoagulation).

■ 免疫グロブリンが効かない場合はステロイドの点滴を行うこともあります．

If immunoglobulin is not effective, intravenous steroid may be given.

■ 通常は2～3週間で退院となりますが，心臓の合併症を確認するため，退院後も心臓超音波検査を何度か行う必要があります．

Usually it requires hospitalization for 2 to 3 weeks. To check if there is any heart complication, follow up with echocardiogram is needed periodically.

- aspirin　アスピリン
- immunoglobulin　免疫グロブリン

● 薬の副作用　Side effect of medications

■ 免疫グロブリンは，じんましんなどのアレルギー反応を起こすことがあります．

Immunogloblin may cause allergic reaction such as rash.

■ また献血から作られる血液製剤であるためウイルス感染を起こすこともありますが，極めてまれです．

Immunogloblin is a blood derivative produced from donated blood. In extremely rare cases, if the donated blood is contaminated, it may cause viral infection.

保護者へのアドバイス　Advice to parents

★ 治療のゴールは冠動脈にコブを作らないことです．

Treatment goal is to prevent aneurysms formed in the coronary arteries.

★ 治療により多くは完治します．

In most cases full recovery can be expected.

Part 4　4. 病名を英語で説明する：英語を使った小児科診療・病名編

19　てんかん
Epilepsy

● こんな病気　Overview

- けいれん発作をくり返す脳の病気です．
  Epilepsy is a brain disorder involving repeated seizures.
- 脳に火花を起こす部分があり，一旦発火すると電気が脳内に広がってけいれんを起こします．
  There are abnormal sparks in brain wiring. Seizures are caused by abnormally excited electrical signals spread in the brain.
- てんかんは 100 人に 1 人の割合で起こりますので，めずらしい病気ではありません．
  Epilepsy occurs 1 in 100 people. This is not an uncommon disorder.
- 子どものてんかんは，適切な治療により 70〜80％ は完治するといわれています．
  Full recovery can be expected with appropriate treatment in 70 to 80% of children with epilepsy.

● 原　因　Cause

- けいれんを起こしやすい体質と，何らかの理由で脳にダメージが起こった場合の 2 つの原因があります．
  There are two causes : idiopathic cause and the result from brain damage.
- 後者には，①生まれつき（遺伝や脳の奇形など），②生まれる前後（仮死状態など），③生まれたあと（頭のけがや脳の病気など）があります．
  Brain damage is : 1) congenital (genetics, malformation in the brain).
  2) the injury occurred during the birth (fetal distress), 3) the injury occurred after the birth (by head injury or brain disease).

● 症　状　Symptom

- 突然意識がなくなり，白目をむき，顔色が真っ青になり，手足が硬くなったりガクガクふるわせたりするけいれんが起こります．
  Patients who are having seizures lose consciousness suddenly, roll their eyes back, and get pale. Muscle rigidity and violent muscle contractions in the extremities occur.
- 顔や手足の一部分だけがピクピクする場合や，意識がはっきりしている場合，短時間ボーッとするだけの場合もあります．
  Episode may involve only twitching in the face or part of extremities. When the patients are conscious, the lack of awareness of surroundings only occurs for a short period of time.

● 検　査　Test

- 血液や尿検査，頭の CT や MRI，脳波検査などで診断します．
  Samples from blood and urine, head CT and MRI, and EEG are used to diagnose.

19. てんかん　Epilepsy

●治療　Treatment

■抗てんかん薬（けいれん止め）を内服し，脳内の火花を抑えます．
Oral anticonvulsants are taken to suppress sparks in the brain.

■一般的に2回目のけいれん発作を起こした場合に治療を開始しますが，状況によっては1回目のけいれん発作から開始する場合もあります．
In general, treatment starts from the second episode of seizure. Depending on the condition, treatment may start after the first episode.

■最後のけいれん発作から2～4年間は治療を続け，脳波検査で薬の中止を判断します．
Treatment continues 2 to 4 years after the last episode. Ending the seizure medications is determined depending on the result of EEG.

■もともとの原因によっては，なかなか薬を中止できない場合もあります．
Certain types of epilepsy may need long term medication.

- Oral anticonvulsants　抗てんかん薬

●薬の副作用　Side effect of medications

■眠気やふらつき，アレルギー反応（発疹など）を起こす場合があります．
They may cause drowsiness, dizziness, and allergic reactions (rash).

■肝臓・腎臓の疲れや，血液中の白血球・赤血球などが減ってしまうこともあるため，定期的な血液や尿検査が必要です．
Fatigue in the liver and kidney, reduction in the number of white and red blood cells may occur. Regular blood and urine tests are required.

- Fatigue in the liver　肝臓の疲れ
- Fatigue in the kidney　腎臓の疲れ
- White blood cells　白血球
- Red blood cells　赤血球

保護者へのアドバイス　Advice to parents

★睡眠不足や疲労時に発作が起こりやすくなるため，普段から規則正しい日常生活が大切です．
Some factors such as lack of sleep and fatigue can increase the risk of a seizure. Your children need to keep well-regulated life.

★抗てんかん薬を急に中止すると大きな発作が突然再発する場合があるため，飲み忘れや自己判断での中止は避けましょう．
When you stop taking anticonvulsants suddenly, an intense seizure may recur. Avoid skipping dosages or stopping medications without your doctors' instruction.

20 先天性心疾患
Congenital heart disease

●こんな病気　Overview

■ 何らかの原因で生まれつき（先天性）持っている心臓病で，約 100 人に 1 人の割合で起こります．
This is a heart disease present at birth (congenital) and it occurs 1 in 100 people.

■ 心臓は，4 つの部屋が壁や弁（ドア）によって仕切られています．
それぞれの部屋は大きな血管で全身や肺とつながっています．
Heart is divided into four chambers by walls and valves (doors).
Each chamber is connected to the whole body and lungs by arteries and veins.

■ 体中を流れる血液は，肺で酸素を受け取り，一旦心臓に戻った後に全身に送られます．
Blood circulates in the body receives oxygen in the lungs and returns to the heart. The heart pumps the blood to the whole body.

■ 内臓などに酸素を渡し，再び心臓に戻ってきた後，肺に送られまた酸素を受け取ります．
Blood brings in oxygen including to the organs and returns to the heart. Then the heart pushes the blood to the lungs and the whole process starts over.

■ 先天性心疾患は，心臓の部屋の壁に穴があいているもの・心臓弁の故障・血管の異常など，約 50 種類もの病気があります．
また，軽いものから重いものまで，生まれてすぐに緊急手術が必要なものから大人になって気付かれるものまで様々です．
There are about 50 different kinds of congenital heart disease : holes in the heart chambers walls, defect of the valves, abnormalities in blood vessels, etc.
Symptoms vary from mild to severe : emergency surgical repair might be required right after the birth. The defects can be detected in much later in adult life.

●原　因　Cause

■ 多くは原因不明ですが，母親の喫煙，薬剤・アルコール摂取，風疹などのウイルス感染，染色体異常などの影響を受けることもあります．
Causes of most congenital heart disease are not identified, however, factors such as mother's smoking habits, drug and alcohol use, viral infection such as rubella, and chromosomal abnormalities may increase the risks of getting it.

●症　状　Symptom

■ チアノーゼ：体の酸素が足りないため，顔色が悪くなり唇も紫色になります．
Cyanosis : blue and purple discoloration on the face and lips due to lack of oxygen

■ 心不全：十分な血液を全身に送り出せないために，呼吸が苦しくなります．
Heart failure : difficulty in breathing due to a pump fails to maintain the circulation of blood to the whole body.

20. 先天性心疾患　Congenital heart disease

■この2つの症状によりミルクも飲みにくくなり，体重が増えなくなります．
Because of these two symptoms, the infants with the defect have difficulties with taking milk and gaining weight.
・Cyanosis　チアノーゼ
・Heart failure　心不全

●検　査　Test
■心電図・心臓超音波検査・胸部エックス線・CT・MRI・血液検査・心臓カテーテル検査などで診断します．
ECG, echocardiography, chest x-ray, CT and MRI, blood test, and cardiac catheterization are done to diagnose.
- □心電図　ECG
- □心臓超音波検査　Echocardiography
- □胸部エックス線　Chest X-ray
- □CT　CT scan
- □MRI　MRI (magnetic resonanoe imaging)
- □血液検査　Blood test
- □心臓カテーテル検査　Cardiac catheterization

●治　療　Treatment
■病気の種類・程度により，内服や注射などの薬物治療，手術，心臓カテーテル治療が行われます．
Depending on the types and degrees of severity of the congenital heart disease, oral medications or injections, surgeries, and cardiac catheterization therapy are administered.

保護者へのアドバイス　Advice to parents

★ミルクを飲む時に苦しそうな場合は，1回の量を少なめにしてこまめにあげるのがよいでしょう．
If your children have a difficulty with swallowing milk, give out small amount at a time and more often.

★かぜを引き金に病気が悪化する場合がありますので，うがいや手洗いなど家族みんながかぜにかからないように心がけましょう．
Cold may trigger the symptoms to worsen. All family members need to take precautions not to catch a cold by washing hands and gurgle.

★聴診で心雑音があると言われた場合，害のないものと病気が疑われるものがありますので，必要に応じて検査を受けることになります．
When a heart murmur is found by stethoscopy, it can be an innocent murmur or diseases might be associated with it：further testing is required.

★代表的な先天性心疾患　　Typical congenital heart disease
・チアノーゼがないもの：心房中隔欠損症・心室中隔欠損症・房室中隔欠損症・動脈管開存症．
　Non-cyanotic：atrial septal defect, ventricular septal defect, atrioventricular septal defect, patent ductus arteriosus.
・チアノーゼがあるもの：ファロー四徴症・完全大血管転位症・両大血管右室起始症など．
　Cyanotic：Tetralogy of Fallot, complete transposition of great arteries, double-outlet right ventricle.
・(例)心室中隔欠損症　　Example：Ventricular septal defect

★左右の心室の間にある「心室中隔」という壁に穴があいている病気です．
　This is a defect with holes in the wall, "ventricular septum," that separates the right and left ventricles.

★先天性心疾患のうちもっとも多い病気で，約6割を占めるといわれています．
　This is the most common congenital heart disease. It accounts for about 60% of cases.

★となりの部屋から血液が乱入してくるために血液の通り道が交通渋滞となり，心臓や肺に負担がかかることがあります．
　When the amount of blood crossing the defect is high, blood vessels are congested and causes distress to the heart and lungs.

★穴が小さい場合はいずれ自然に閉じることもありますが，穴が大きく症状が強い場合は，一般的に手術で穴を閉じます．
　When holes are small, they may close on their own. When the holes are large and symptoms are severe, surgical repair is needed.

21 気管支ぜんそく
Bronchial asthma

Part 4　4．病名を英語で説明する：英語を使った小児科診療・病名編

● こんな病気　Overview

■ 気管支ぜんそくとは，発作性に喘鳴（ゼーゼー，ヒューヒュー）を伴う呼吸困難をくり返す病気です．
Bronchial Asthma is an illness with periodic attacks of stridor (wheezing) that may cause respiratory distress.
・Wheezing　ゼーゼー，ヒューヒュー（した咳）

■ ぜんそくの子どもでは，気道の炎症がつねに起こっています．
Children with asthma have chronic inflammation in the bronchial tubes.

■ ぜんそくの多くは，1〜2歳で発症します．
In most cases it appears by 1 to 2 years of age.

■ 2歳までに60％の子どもが発症し，3歳までに80％の子どもが発症します．
60% of the cases appear by 2 years of age and 80% by 3 years of age.

● 原　因　Cause

■ 気管支ぜんそくは，遺伝的な原因と環境的な原因が組み合わさって発症します．
It is a combination of hereditary and environmental factors.

■ 遺伝的な原因とは，本人の体質です．
Hereditary means disease caused by genetic factors.

■ 環境的な原因には，ダニなどのアレルゲン，風邪，タバコなどの空気の汚れ，天候などがあります．
Environmental causes are allergens such as ticks, common cold, air pollution that come from smoke and other sources, and climates.

● 症　状　Symptom

■ 気管支ぜんそくの症状として，喘鳴（ゼーゼー，ヒューヒュー）や咳，胸のペコペコした動き，息苦しさ，などがみられます．
Stridor (wheezing), coughs, see-saw motions in the chest from labored breathing, and difficulty in breathing are observed.

■ 症状は，その時の状態によって，軽いものから重いものまであります．
Symptoms vary from mild to severe, depending on the patient's condition.

■ 症状が軽ければ，話すことができ，食事や睡眠ができます．
Symptoms can be mild with no difficulties in talking, eating, and sleeping.

■ 症状が重いと，話すこともできず，食事や睡眠もできなくなります．
Symptoms can be severe enough to obstruct patients with talking, eating, and sleeping.

● 検　査　Test

■ 気管支ぜんそくの診断には，検査は重要ではありません．病歴や症状から，診断します．

病名カテゴリー別
呼吸器
循環器
神経・精神
アレルギー
消化器
泌尿器
外傷
感染症
内分泌・代謝
耳・鼻・咽喉
皮膚

To diagnose bronchial asthma, tests are not important but can be used in certain circumstances. It can be diagnosed from medical history and symptoms.

☐血液検査（アレルギー検査）　Blood test (Allergy test)
☐エックス線検査　X-ray test
☐肺機能検査　Pulmonary Function Test

●治　療　Treatment

1．気管支ぜんそく発作のコントロール　Control of asthma

■気道の炎症をおさえ，発作をコントロールすることが大切です．
It is important to reduce the inflammation in the bronchial tubes and control the attacks.

■薬を始める時は，発作がどれくらいの期間に，どれくらいの回数起こっているのか，チェックします．
Before starting medications, the duration and frequency of asthma attacks should be checked.

■コントロールする薬には，アレルギーの薬，気管支を拡げる薬，ステロイドの薬などがあります．
Medications for sustained control or quick relief of symptoms include medications for allergy, bronchodilator, and steroids.

■治療を行って，日常生活が普通に送れるようになることが目標です．
Goal is to have a full quality of life with treatment.

2．発作時の薬　Medication for acute attacks

■発作が起こった時は，気管支を拡げる薬を吸入します．
When acute attack occurs, inhale medication to dilate bronchi.

■吸入で発作が良くならない時は，点滴が必要になります．
If inhaler does not improve the asthma symptoms, medication through IV is needed.

3．環境的な原因の除去　Removal of environmental triggers.

■原因と考えられるもの（アレルゲン，タバコの煙など）を，取り除くことが大切です．
It is important to avoid triggers (allergen and smoke, etc).

●薬の副作用　Side effect of medications

1．眠気　Drowsiness

■アレルギーの薬で，眠気がみられることがあります．
Drowsiness may occur with allergy medications.

■ただし，最近の薬は，あまり眠くならないようになっています．
Newly approved medications cause less drowsiness.

2．手の震え，動悸（胸のドキドキ）　Tremor in hands, palpitation (heart pounding)

■気管支を拡げる薬で，手が震えたり，動悸がみられることがあります．
Bronchodilator may cause tremor in hands and palpitation.

21. 気管支ぜんそく　Bronchial asthma

3．口の中の症状　Symptoms in the mouth
■ステロイドの吸入では，のどの刺激感，声のかすれ，などがみられることがあります．
When steroid is inhaled, it may irritate the throat or cause hoarseness.

4．興奮，不眠　Hyperactivity, insomnia
■気管支を拡げる薬の量が多いと，興奮や不眠がみられることがあります．
High dosage of medication to dilate bronchi may cause hyperactivity and insomnia.

5．消化器の症状　Symptoms in digestive system
■気管支を拡げる薬の量が多いと，腹痛や吐き気，嘔吐がみられることがあります．
High dosage of medication to dilate bronchi may cause abdominal pain, nausea, vomiting.

6．けいれん　Convulsion
■気管支を拡げる薬の量が多いと，まれにけいれんが起こることがあります．
High dosage of medication to dilate bronchi may cause convulsion but this happens rarely.

7．その他　Others
■ステロイドは，決められた量を守って飲めば，全身の副作用はほとんどありません．
When steroid is taken as prescribed, there are few side effects on the body.

保護者へのアドバイス　Advice to parents

★ぜんそくの薬は，毎日続けることが大切です．
It is important to take medications every day.

★子どもや親の判断で，薬を減らしたり，中止したりしないようにしましょう．
Do not reduce the dosage or stop taking medications without your doctors' instruction.

★発作のない状態が5年続けば，ぜんそくは治ったと判断します．
When asthma attack does not occur for 5 years, it is considered that asthma has been cured.

病名カテゴリー別
呼吸器
循環器
神経・精神
アレルギー
消化器
泌尿器
外傷
感染症
内分泌・代謝
耳・鼻・咽喉
皮膚

Part 4

4. 病名を英語で説明する：英語を使った小児科診療・病名編

22 アトピー性皮膚炎
Atopic dermatitis

●こんな病気　Overview

■アトピー性皮膚炎とは，痒みのある湿疹が悪くなったり，良くなったりをくり返す病気です．

Atopic dermatitis is a chronic skin problem with itching eczema, which repeatedly gets better or worse over time.

■アトピー性皮膚炎では，皮膚の乾燥とバリア機能の低下があります．

The affected skin areas appear dry and sensitive.

■そこへ，いろいろな刺激やアレルギー反応が加わって症状がでます．

Symptoms flare by certain irritants and allergic reaction.

■多くは乳幼児期に発症しますが，それ以降でも発症します．

Most cases appear in infants but it may appear in the later life.

●原　因　Cause

■アトピー性皮膚炎は，遺伝的な原因と環境的な原因が組み合わさって発症します．

It is a combination of hereditary and environmental factors.

■遺伝的な原因とは，本人の体質です．

Hereditary means disease caused by genetic factors.

■環境的な原因には，ダニなどのアレルゲン，食物，洗剤など，たくさんありますが，病気を悪くする原因は人それぞれです．

Environmental factors include allergens such as ticks, food, detergent, etc. Which factor worsens the symptoms depend on the patient.

●症　状　Symptom

■アトピー性皮膚炎の症状として，痒みのある湿疹がみられます．

Itching eczema appears as a typical symptom of atopic dermatitis.

■乳児期の湿疹は，口のまわりや頬，その他の顔，頭，耳，肘や膝の内側にみられます．

In babies, eczema appears around the mouth, cheeks, other parts of the face, head, ears, and inner side of elbows and knees.

■幼児期〜学童の湿疹は，体(とくに背中)や，肘や膝の内側にみられます．

In infants to schoolchildren, eczema is seen on the torso (especially back) and inner side of elbows and knees.

■思春期の湿疹は，額や首，肘や膝の内側にみられます．

In puberty, eczema is seen on the temple, neck, and inner side of elbows and knees.

■一般的に，冬〜春にかけて悪化します．

In general it is worse from winter to spring.

22. アトピー性皮膚炎　Atopic dermatitis

●検　査　Test

■アトピー性皮膚炎の診断には，検査は重要ではありません．病歴や症状から診断します．
To diagnose atopic dermatitis, tests are not important but can be used in certain circumstances. Medical history and symptoms are used to diagnose.
　□血液検査　Blood test
　□アレルギー検査　Allergy test

●治　療　Treatment

1．スキンケア　Skincare
■皮膚を清潔に保つために，お風呂やシャワーで体をきちんと洗います．
To keep skin hygienic, use bathtub or take shower.
■お風呂の温度が高いと，痒みがでますので，高い温度を避けます．
Hot water triggers itching. Avoid using very hot water.
■刺激の少ない石けんで軽く洗います．
Use mild soap and wash lightly.
■保湿薬を1日2回（朝とお風呂あがり），塗ります．
Apply moisturizer twice a day (morning and after the bath).

2．痒み止め　Medication to relieve itching
■痒みがある場合は，痒みを抑える薬を使います．
When it gets itchy, medication to relieve it is used.

3．塗り薬　Ointment
■症状が強い時には，ステロイドの塗り薬を使います．
When the symptoms are intense, steroid ointment is prescribed.
■ステロイド以外の塗り薬として，免疫をおさえる塗り薬があります．
Besides steroid ointment, immunosuppressant ointment is available.

●薬の副作用　Side effect of medications

1．眠気　Drowsiness
■痒み止めの飲み薬で，眠気を感じることがあります．
Oral medication to reduce itching may cause drowsiness.
■ただし，最近の薬は，あまり眠くならないようになっています．
Newly approved medications cause less drowsiness.

2．かぶれ　Rash
■炎症をおさえる塗り薬で，ステロイドや免疫をおさえる薬が入っていないものでは，かぶれがみられることがあります．
Anti inflammatory ointment without steroid or immunosuppressant may cause rash.

3．皮膚の萎縮，小さな血管の拡張　Atrophy of skin, dilation of capillary
■ステロイドを長い間大量に使用すると，皮膚が薄くなり，赤くなることがあります．
Long term steroid use may cause the skin get thinner and red.

4．熱感，痛み　Heat, pain
■免疫をおさえる塗り薬を使用すると，塗り始めて数日間，塗った部位がほってたり，ヒリ

ヒリすることがあります．

Immunosuppressant ointment may cause flush or soreness on the applied area in the first few days.

■ しかし，症状がよくなるとともに，ほてりやヒリヒリも消えていきます．

When the symptoms get better, flush or soreness will go away.

・Soreness　ヒリヒリ（した痛み）

保護者へのアドバイス　Advice to parents

★アトピー性皮膚炎は，治りにくい病気です．時間をかけて，ゆっくり治していくことが大切です．

Atopic dermatitis is difficult to cure. It is important to be patient.

★子どもや親の判断で，薬を減らしたり，中止したりしないようにしましょう．

Do not reduce or stop medications without your doctor's instruction.

★塗り薬の使い方として，フィンガーティップユニット（FTU）があります．これは，大人の人差し指の第一関節の長さ（約0.5g）を出した場合，大人の手のひら2枚くらいの広さの患部に塗るのが適量という考え方です．（参考：43ページ）

To apply ointment, finger-tip unit (FTU) can be used to measure the amount. If ointment expressed from a tube as same length as from the tip to the first crease in adult index finger (about 0.5 g), it is appropriate to treat an area of skin twice the size of the flat of an adult's hand with the fingers together. (Reference：43 page)

23 食物アレルギー
Food allergies

● こんな病気　Overview

- 食物アレルギーとは，原因食物を食べた後に，免疫学的に体にとって悪い症状が起きる病気です．
  Food allergies are a bad immunological reaction caused by exposure to specific food.
- 一般的に食物アレルギーは，原因食物を食べて 2 時間以内に症状が現れます．
  In general, symptoms appear within 2 hours after eating.
- その他に，アトピー性皮膚炎が関係する食物アレルギーや，運動をすることによって症状が現れる食物アレルギーもあります．
  There are food allergies related to atopic dermatitis. Some food allergies induced by exercises.
- 食物アレルギーは，0 歳にもっとも多くみられ，その後，年齢とともに減っていきます．
  It is most common in infants younger than 12 months of age and often they outgrow the allergies.
- 食物アレルギーは，3 歳までに 7 割の子どもが発症し，8 歳までに 8 割の子どもが発症します．
  70% of the cases appear by 3 years of age and 80% appear by 8 years of age.
  - Specific food　原因食物
  - Atopic dermatitis　アトピー性皮膚炎

● 原　因　Cause

- 食物アレルギーの原因は，乳幼児では卵，牛乳，小麦が多くみられます．
  Eggs, milk, and flour are the most common source of food allergies in infants.
- 学童では甲殻類，小麦，果実が多くみられます．
  Shellfish, flour, and fruits are the common source of food allergies in school children.

● 症　状　Symptom

- 食物アレルギーでは，頻度の多い順に，皮膚，呼吸器，粘膜，消化器の症状がみられます．
  The most frequent allergic reactions in order of prevalence：they appear to the skin, respiratory systems, mucus membranes, and digestive systems.
- 具体的には，皮膚ならじんましんや湿疹，呼吸器ならくしゃみや鼻水，粘膜なら目や口の症状，消化器なら下痢など，がみられます．
  If it affects the skin, hives and eczema may develop, if it affects the respiratory system, it may cause sneezing and runny nose. If it affects mucous membranes, the reaction occurs in the eyes and mouth. Diarrhea would be induced if it affects the digestive systems.
- 時にショック症状（意識障害や血圧低下など）がみられます．
  Severe shock reaction may occur (disturbance of consciousness and drop in blood pressure).
- ショックは，原因食物を食べてから数分以内に起こることが多く，口やのどの腫れ・痒み，

吐き気，嘔吐などがみられます．
Swelling in the mouth and throat, itching, nausea, and vomiting are common shock reactions that occur within minutes after exposure to the food.
- Hives　じんましん
- Eczema　湿疹
- Sneezing　くしゃみ
- Runny nose　鼻水
- Mucous membrane　粘膜
- Diarrhea　下痢

●検　査　Test

■問診や血液検査，皮膚テストの結果を参考にし，最終的には食物除去試験・負荷試験によって判定します．
History taking, blood and skin tests are used. The final diagnosis is made by elimination diet and food tolerance test.
□血液検査　Blood test
□皮膚テスト　Skin test
□食物除去試験　Elimination Diet
□食物負荷試験　Food tolerance test

●治　療　Treatment

1．原因除去　Dietary avoidance
■原因となる食物を除去します．
Remove the identified food that causes allergic reaction
■不必要なものまで除去しないようにします．
Try not to remove other food. Only remove the allergen.

2．調理法の工夫　Preparation
■原因となる食物のなかには，加熱や加工によって食べることができるものもあります．
Some food allergens can be tolerated by heating or processing.
■ただし，ショックを起こした食物は，加工品でも除去します．
If the food causes shock reaction, eliminate it even when it is processed.

3．代わりになる食品　Substitute
■除去する食物の代わりになる食品を探し，栄養が不足しないようにします．
Use substitutes for the allergen to supplement nutrition.

4．アレルギーの薬　Medication
■アレルギーの薬を補助的に使うことがあります．
Allergy medications might be used as adjuvant.

5．ショックの治療　Treatment for shock reaction
■ショック症状がみられた場合は，ショックの治療を行います．
Specific treatment is need when shock reaction occurs.

23. 食物アレルギー　Food allergies

6. 除去食の解除　Removal of dietary restrictions

■原因食物は，年齢とともに食べることができるようになることもあるので，徐々に解除していきます．

Since children may outgrow the allergy, gradually expose them to the food.

●薬の副作用　Side effect of medications

1．消化器の症状　Digestive system

■アレルギーの薬で，下痢や食欲不振，腹痛などがみられることがあります．

Allergy medications might cause diarrhea, loss of appetite, and abdominal pain.

2．発疹　Rash

■アレルギーの薬で，発疹がみられることがあります．

Allergy medications might cause rash.

保護者へのアドバイス　Advice to parents

★食物の除去は，医師と相談し，必要最小限にしましょう．

Consult with your doctors when you remove the food allergen from your children's diet and make the nutritional impact minimal.

★赤ちゃんでアレルギー体質が疑われる場合，離乳食を遅らせる必要はありません．アレルギーが起こりにくいものから始めましょう．

When your babies are suspected to have food allergies, you do not need to delay in giving them solid food. Start with food less likely to cause allergy.

Part 4

24 じんましん
Hives, Urticaria

● こんな病気　Overview

- じんましんとは，突然，皮膚の一部が赤くくっきりと盛り上がり，しばらくすると消えてしまう病気です．
  Hives are outbreak of red bumps on the skin that appear suddenly and fade after a while.
- 多くは痒みを伴いますが，チクチクとした痒みに似た感じや，焼けるような感じを伴うこともあります．
  They usually cause itching and may cause stinging and or burning as well.
- 虫刺されに似ていますが，虫刺されは，ひっかいているうちに表面がジクジクしたりします．じんましんでは，それがありません．
  They look like insect stings but when scratched, insect stings may become oozy. This does not happen with hives.
- じんましんは，年齢に関係なく発症します．
  Hives appear in all ages.
  - Insect sting　虫刺され
  - Oozy　ジクジク（ただれる）

● 原　因　Cause

- アレルギーが原因のこともありますし，アレルギー以外の原因のこともあります．
  Both allergic reaction and other factors can cause hives.
- アレルギーの原因として，飲み物や食べ物，薬品，植物，昆虫の毒などの接触，などがあります．
  Allergic reaction causes include food, medicines, plants, and contact with insect poisons.
- アレルギー以外の原因として，物理的な刺激やストレス，などがあります．
  In additions to allergic reaction, hives can be caused by physical stimulation and stress.
  - Food　飲み物や食べ物
  - Medicines　薬品
  - Plant　植物
  - Insect poison　昆虫の毒
  - Physical stimulation　物理的な刺激
  - Stress　ストレス

● 症　状　Symptom

- 普通，発疹は30分〜2時間で消えるか，別の場所に移動します．
  Usually eruptions last for 30 minutes to 2 hours or move to different parts of the skin.
- なかには，半日から1日くらいまで発疹が続くことがあります．
  Some last for half a day to 1 day.
- 症状が激しい場合には，次々と新しい発疹が現れ，つねに発疹が現れているようにみえる

24. じんましん　Hives, Urticaria

こともあります．

When its symptoms are severe, new eruptions break out one after another. Eruptions can appear constantly somewhere on the body.

■発疹の大きさは，1〜2 mm 程度のものから，手足全体位のものまでいろいろです．

Hives vary in size：from 1-2 mm to the size of the whole hand or foot.

■形はいろいろですが，その形に意味はありません．

Hives vary in shape but shapes do not mean anything.

●検　査　Test

■検査をしても，原因が見つからないことがほとんどです．食物アレルギーが疑われる場合は，血液検査で原因がわかることもあります．

Tests cannot identify the cause in most cases. In case of food allergy, cause can be found by blood test.

　□血液検査　　Blood test
　□皮膚テスト　Skin test

●治　療　Treatment

1．原因の除去　Removal of the triggers

■じんましんの原因と考えられるものを避けます．

Avoid the factors that cause hives.

■飲み物や食べ物が原因と考えられる場合は，不必要なものまで除去しないようにします．

When a specific food is the cause, try not to eliminate food other than allergen.

2．患部の治療　Treatment for the affected areas

■患部をかくと，痒みが強くなるので，できるだけかかないようにします．

Try not to scratch. Scratching will worsen itching.

■患部は温めないようにします．

Avoid heating the affected areas.

■痒みが強い場合は，冷たいもので冷やすと，痒みが和らぎます．

When itching is intense, cooling down the areas will ease itching.

3．アレルギーの薬　Allergy medications

■痒みがある場合は，痒みをおさえる薬を使います．

When it gets itchy, medications are used to ease it.

4．ステロイド　Steroid

■症状が強い場合には，ステロイドを使うことがあります．

When symptoms are intense, steroid may be used.

●薬の副作用　Side effect of medications

1．眠気　Drowsiness

■アレルギーの薬で，眠気がみられることがあります．

Allergy medications may cause drowsiness.

■ただし，最近の薬は，あまり眠くならないようになっています．

Newly approved medications cause less drowsiness.

2．その他　Others

■ステロイドは，短い間しか使わないので，副作用はほとんどありません．
Side effect is minimal with short term use of steroid.

保護者へのアドバイス　Advice to parents

★アレルギーが原因でショック症状が起こることあり，その時の皮膚症状として，じんましんが現れることがあります．
Allergy may cause a shock reaction. One of the symptoms of a shock reaction is hives appearing on the skin.

★呼吸器の症状（声のかすれ，息苦しさ），循環器の症状（唇や顔色が悪い）などの症状を認める場合は，すぐに病院を受診しましょう．
When you see reactions in your children's respiratory system (hoarseness, difficulty in breathing) or circulatory system (pale lips and face), call an ambulance.

Part 4 — 25. 糖尿病
Diabetes mellitus

4. 病名を英語で説明する：英語を使った小児科診療・病名編

● こんな病気　Overview

- 糖尿病とは，血液中の糖が正常量を超えて増えたため，いろいろな症状や合併症が現れてくる病気です．
  Diabetes is a disease develops when blood sugar level is higher than normal and it causes symptoms and complications.
- インスリン（血糖を下げるホルモン）が絶対的に不足することによって起こる糖尿病を，1型糖尿病といいます．
  Type I diabetes is caused when insulin (hormone lowers the blood sugar) secretion is very little or none.
- 肥満などの生活習慣病によって起こる糖尿病を，2型糖尿病といいます．
  Type II diabetes is caused by lifestyle-related illness such as obesity.
- 最近では，生活習慣の変化によって，2型糖尿病の子どもが増えてきています．
  Because of a change in life style, more children are now diagnosed with type II diabetes.
  - Type Ⅰ diabetes　1型糖尿病
  - Type Ⅱ diabetes　2型糖尿病

● 原　因　Cause

- 1型糖尿病の原因は，インスリンを分泌する細胞が壊れることです．
  Cause of type I is when cells which secrete insulin are destroyed.
- インスリンを分泌する細胞が壊れる原因は，まだはっきりしていません．
  Exact cause of why these cells are destroyed has not been identified.
- 2型糖尿病の原因は，インスリンの分泌が低下したり，反応が悪くなることです．
  Cause of type II is the secretion of insulin is decreased or not used effectively.

● 症　状　Symptom

- 糖尿病の症状として，高血糖になると血液が濃くなります．
  それを薄めるために水分を必要とするため，口が渇くようになります．
  When blood sugar is high, blood gets thick.
  To make the blood thinner, more fluid is needed and this causes excessive thirst.
- 体が，多量の水分といっしょに糖を尿中に出そうとするため，多尿になります．
  The body tries to get rid of glucose by excreting it as urine. Therefore frequent urination occurs.
- 糖をエネルギーとして使えず，脂肪が分解されるため，病気が進行すると体重が減ります．
  Since the body cannot use glucose as a source of energy, when the disease progress body fat is used instead which causes weight loss.

■病気の進行が遅いと，症状がないため，学校の尿検査でみつかることがあります．
When this disease progresses slowly no symptoms appear. Urine test at school may detect it.

■病気が進行すると，脂肪が分解され，ケトアシドーシス*という状態になり，呼吸が速くなり，脱水がみられます．
When the disease progresses further fat is broken down and a serious condition called ketoacidosis develops. Rapid breathing and dehydration appear.

●検　査　Test

■糖尿病の診断には，血液検査とブドウ糖の負荷試験を行います．
To diagnose, blood test and glucose tolerance test are performed.

　　□血液検査　Blood test
　　□尿検査　Urine test
　　□ブドウ糖負荷試験　Glucose tolerance test

●治　療　Treatment

1．インスリン　Insulin

■1型糖尿病では，インスリンを毎日注射して，血糖をコントロールします．
In type I diabetes, inject insulin everyday to control blood sugar.

■1型糖尿病では，生きている間，インスリンの注射が必要となります．
In type I diabetes, insulin injection is required for the entire life.

■2型糖尿病では，インスリンの注射はあまり行いません．
In type II diabetes, insulin injection is not often used.

2．食事療法　Diet

■肥満による2型糖尿病では，適切な食事の管理を行います．
When obesity is the cause of type II diabetes, management of appropriate diet is used.

3．運動療法　Exercise

■肥満による2型糖尿病では，適切な運動を行います．
When obesity is the cause of type II diabetes, appropriate exercise is used.

4．血糖を下げる飲み薬　Oral medication to lower blood sugar

■2型糖尿病で，食事の管理と運動で血糖がコントロールできない場合は，血糖を下げる飲み薬を使います．
If blood glucose level is not controlled with diet and exercise in type II diabetes, oral hypoglycemic agent is used.

■1型糖尿病では，この飲み薬は使いません．
This agent is not used for type I diabetes.

---

*ケトアシドーシス…脂肪がドンドン分解されると，ケトン体という物質がたまり，アシドーシス（血液が酸性に傾く状態）となります．
Ketoacidosis…When fat is broken down, ketone bodies are deposited in the bloodstream and it causes acidosis（the blood becomes more acidic）.

25. 糖尿病　Diabetes mellitus

●薬の副作用　Side effect of medications
【低血糖　Hypoglycemia】
■インスリン注射や血糖を下げる飲み薬で，血糖が下がりすぎることがあります．
Insulin injection and oral hypoglycemic agent may cause hypoglycemia.

---　保護者へのアドバイス　Advice to parents　---

★1型糖尿病の子どもは，体調が悪くて食事が食べられない時にも，インスリン注射が必要となります．
Children with type I diabetes need insulin injection even when they feel sick and cannot take meals.

★その時，どれくらいのインスリンを注射すればいいのか，あらかじめ主治医の先生から聞いておきましょう．
Get your doctors' instruction in advance about how much insulin should be administered in such case.

★冷汗や動悸（胸のドキドキ），空腹感などの低血糖発作が現れたら，急いで糖分を与えましょう．
When your children show hypoglycemia attack, such as cold sweat and palpitation (heart pounding), or hunger, give them sugar quickly.

★血糖値をきちんとコントロールしないと，血管がもろくなり，発症から10年前後で，いろいろな合併症があらわれてきます
If you do not maintain control of your children's blood glucose level, the veins get fragile and numerous complications develop in 10 years.

Part 4　4. 病名を英語で説明する：英語を使った小児科診療・病名編

26　肥　満
Obesity

●こんな病気　Overview

■肥満とは，脂肪が一定以上に多くなった病気のことです．
Obesity is a condition having body fat above a certain level.

■食生活の変化やテレビゲームの普及など，子どもを取り巻く環境が変わり，子どもの肥満が増えてきています．
Childhood obesity is increasing due to a change in diet and widespread use of TV games.

■肥満傾向は，男子に多くみられ，9〜11歳以降に多くみられます．
Tendency to be obese is more common in boys, especially after 9 to 11 years of age.

■赤ちゃんの肥満は，そのまま幼児になっても続くことはありません．
Obesity in babies does not pass onto childhood.

●原　因　Cause

■肥満の原因は，とくに病気のない単純性肥満と，病気が背景にある症候性肥満の2つがあります．
There are two causes：simple obesity with no disease associated with it and symptomatic obesity associated with disease.

■単純性肥満の原因には，遺伝的な原因や生活習慣，環境があげられます．
In simple obesity, causes can be genetic, life style, and environment.

■症候性肥満の原因は，ホルモンの病気や，染色体の異常のことがあります．
In symptomatic obesity, hormonal disease or chromosome abnormality would be the cause.

・Simple obesity　単純性肥満
・Symptomatic obesity　症候性肥満

●症　状　Symptom

■単純性肥満で，肥満が軽度だと，症状はありません．
With simple and mild obesity, there are no symptoms.

■肥満が高度だと，呼吸が浅くなったり，睡眠時の一時的な呼吸停止がみられます．
When obesity is severe, breathing may be shallow or sleep apnea can develop.

■単純性肥満が続くと，体に脂肪がたまったり，2型糖尿病を発症する危険が高まります．
If simple obesity continues, the risks of storing more fat in the body or developing type II diabetes increase.

■症候性肥満では，その病気に特徴的な症状がみられます．
In symptomatic obesity, symptoms are characteristic to the specific underlying disease associated with it.

26. 肥満　Obesity

● 検　査　Test

■ 肥満の判定は，身長と体重から計算されます．
It is determined by calculation from height and weight.
- □ 身体計測（身長，体重，腹囲）　Physical examination (height, weight, and waist size)
- □ 体脂肪の測定　Body fat measurement
- □ 血圧の測定　Blood pressure measurement
- □ 血液検査　Blood test
- □ 超音波検査　Ultrasound
- □ CT 検査　CT scan

● 治　療　Treatment

■ 単純性肥満の場合，特別な食事療法や運動療法を行なわなくても，身長に見合ったエネルギー摂取と外遊びで十分です．
In case of simple obesity, there is no need to have a special diet and exercise program. Taking appropriate calories for the height and playing outside would be enough.

■ 必要に応じて，食事療法や運動療法を取り入れていきます．
If necessary, use meal plan and exercise program.

1．食事療法　Diet

■ 子どもに必要なエネルギーを計算して，1日の適正なエネルギー量をチェックします．
Calculate how much calories your children need, and check the appropriate calorie intake in a day.

■ エネルギーの計算には，おやつやジュースの量も計算に入れます．
When counting calories intake, snacks and juice must be included.

■ 食事内容は，脂肪を減らし，食物繊維を多く摂るようにします．
Cut down fat and take more fibers.

■ 大人のような厳しい食事制限は，成長を障害する可能性があるので，禁止です．
Heavily restricted diet for adults should be avoided since it prevents healthy growth in your children.

2．運動療法　Therapeutic exercise

■ 脂肪は燃える時にたくさんの酸素を必要とするので，酸素をたっぷり取り込むことのできる有酸素運動を行います．
When fat is burned, so much oxygen is needed. For this reason, aerobic exercise is effective.

3．生活習慣の見直し　Review your life style

■ テレビを見る時間や，ゲームをする時間を減らします．
Reduce time watching TV and playing games.

● 薬の副作用　Side effect of medications

■ 基本的に，肥満で薬を使うことはありません．
Basically, medication is not used to treat obesity.

保護者へのアドバイス　　Advice to parents

★両親，とくに食事を作る親に肥満があると，子どもの肥満はなかなか改善しません．
　If parents, especially the ones who prepare meals are obese, it is difficult to improve obesity in children.

★肥満者のいる家庭では，家族全員の生活を見直しましょう．
　If you have obese family members, check your family lifestyle.

★思春期の肥満や高度の肥満は，治りにくいといわれています．
　Obesity at puberty and severe obesity are difficult to cure.

★思春期に入る前で，肥満が軽いうちに，治療を始めましょう．
　Start the treatment before puberty and while obesity is still mild.

27 外傷・打撲
Trauma, Contusion

● こんな病気　Overview

- 外傷とは，外部から体に受けた傷のことです．
  Trauma is a physical injury due to external action.
- 外傷は，体表面の傷ばかりではなく，骨折や臓器の損傷なども含めます．
  Trauma is injuries not only on the surface of the body but also fractures and injuries of the organs.
- 子どもの頭部外傷では，頭部に作用する力がわずかであっても，出血などの思わぬ事態をひき起こすことがあります．
  In case of head injury in children, even if the impact on the head is minimal, it may cause bleeding and other unexpected conditions.
- 打撲とは，転んだり物にぶつかったりして，傷ができずに皮膚や皮膚の下の組織，筋肉が損傷を受けることです．
  Contusion is not an open wound, it develops when tissues under the skin and muscles get hurt from a bump or fall.

● 原　因　Cause

- 外傷や打撲の原因は，年齢によって異なります．
  子どもの頭部外傷では，転落や転倒，衝突がほとんどです．
  It depends on the age.
  When head injury occurs in children most cases are caused from a fall or a bump.
- 頭部外傷が起こる場所は，0～9歳は家庭内で，10～14歳は学校でもっとも多くみられます．
  The common places where head injury occurs are at home for 0 to 9 years of age and at school for 10 to 14 years of age.
  - Head injury　頭部外傷
  - Fall　転落，転倒
  - Bump　衝突

● 症　状　Symptom

- 外傷の症状として，出血や骨折，臓器の損傷があります．
  Bleeding, fractures, and injuries to the organs are the symptoms of trauma.
- 頭部外傷の症状として，軽度であれば，頭痛や吐き気，嘔吐がみられます．
  Headaches, nausea, and vomiting are the symptoms of mild head injury.
- 頭部外傷が重度であれば，意識障害やけいれんがみられます．
  Disturbance of consciousness and convulsion are the symptoms of severe head injury.
- 打撲の症状として，痛みや腫れ，内出血があります．
  Pain, swelling, and internal bleeding are the symptoms of contusion.
  - Bleeding　出血

- Fracture　骨折
- Injuries to the organ　臓器の損傷
- Headache　頭痛
- Nausea　吐き気
- Vomiting　嘔吐
- Disturbance of consciousness　意識障害
- Convulsion　けいれん

●検　査　Test
■外傷・打撲で，骨折や臓器の出血が疑われる時は，エックス線検査やCT検査が必要となります．

If fracture or injury to the organs is suspected, x-ray (test) or CT scans is needed.
- ☐エックス検査　X-ray
- ☐CT検査　CT scan
- ☐超音波検査　Ultrasound

●治　療　Treatment
【外傷の治療　Trauma】
■まず応急処置をして，すぐに病院を受診します．

Provide first aid and seek medical care at a hospital immediately.

1．意識の確認　Check if the child is conscious or not.

■意識がない，ぐったりしている場合は，気道を確保します．

If the child is unconscious or unresponsive, open the airway.

■呼吸がない場合は，人工呼吸を行います．

If breath is not confirmed, administer artificial respiration.

■脈が触れない場合は，心臓マッサージを行います．

If there is no pulse felt, administer a massage to the heart.

2．止血　Arrest bleeding

■出血がある場合は，まず傷口を直接押さえて止血します．

If the child is bleeding, apply pressure to the open wound directly to stop bleeding.

■それでも拍動する出血がある場合は，傷口よりも心臓に近い場所の動脈を押さえます．

If bleeding continues with pulse, apply pressure to arteries close to the heart.

3．傷口の処置　First aid to a wound

■傷口が汚れている場合は，その周りを水道水で洗い，傷口をきれいなガーゼやタオルでふさぎます．

When the wound is dirty, use tap water to clean the surrounding areas, and dry and cover the area with clean gauze or towel.

4．安静，冷却　Rest, apply ice

■体をむやみに動かさないようにします．

Try not to move the body unless necessary.

■刺さった物がある場合は，抜かないように包帯などで固定します．

27. 外傷・打撲　Trauma, Contusion

When something has pierced the skin, do not remove it but secure it with a dressing.

■患部を冷やします．
Apply ice to the affected area.

【打撲の治療　Contusion】

■基本的な処置は，安静，冷却，圧迫，患部を高く上げる，の４つが大切です．
Basics are：rest, ice, compression, and elevation. These are 4 important procedures.

■内臓や骨の損傷が考えられる場合は，すぐに病院を受診します．
If injuries to the organs or bones are suspected, take the injured child to a hospital immediately.

保護者へのアドバイス　Advice to parents

★子どもはよく転び，頭を打ちつけることがあります．軽度の頭痛や，軽度の吐き気であれば，数時間から１日で症状が落ち着きます．
Children often fall and bump their heads. In case mild headache or nausea appears, symptoms will go away in hours to a day.

★頭部外傷で症状が軽い場合は，急いで病院を受診する必要はありません．しかし，症状が続く時には必ず病院を受診しましょう．
In case of head injury with mild symptoms, you do not need to rush them to hospitals.
However, if symptoms continue, you must seek medical care at a hospital.

Part 4　4. 病名を英語で説明する：英語を使った小児科診療・病名編

28　熱傷
Burns

●こんな病気　Overview

■熱傷とは，火気や高い温度のものに近づいたり，触れたりして起こる病気のことです．
Burns are caused by close contact with fire and high heat objects.

■子どもの皮膚は，大人と比べて薄いので，すぐに深い部分まで熱が伝わります．
Since children's skin is thinner than adults', heat gets penetrates in skin quickly.

■低い温度でも長い時間続くと，湯たんぽやカイロなどによる低温の熱傷が起こります．
Even moderate temperature with exposure for a long time, such as hot water bottle and a pocket heater, can cause burns.

■子どもは，大人と比べて体の水分が多いです．
そのため，重度の場合にショック症状が起こる危険があります．
Children's bodies contain more fluid.
Therefore severe burns may cause shock reactions.

●原　因　Cause

■子どもの熱傷の原因で，多いのは熱湯です．
Common cause of burn in children is hot water.

■その他の原因に，ストーブや花火，炊飯器の蒸気があります．
The next common causes are heater, fireworks, and steam from rice cookers.

●症　状　Symptom

■熱傷の程度によって，I〜III度に分けられます（**表**）．
Burns are categorized as first to third degree burns (Table) depending on the depth of burns.

■I度熱傷の症状は，発赤が主で熱感と痛みがあります．
Symptoms of first degree burns are redness, heat, and pain.

■II度熱傷の症状には，皮膚のはがれや，水ぶくれがあり，強い熱感と痛みがあります．
Symptoms of second degree burns are peeling off the skin, blister, and intense heat and pain.

■III度熱傷の症状では，火気によるものなら皮膚は黒くなり，熱湯や高い温度のものでは皮膚は白くなります．痛みはありません．
Symptoms of third degree burns are if it is caused by fire, the affected skin gets darker and if it is caused by hot water or high heat object, the affected skin gets lighter. There is no pain.

28. 熱傷 Burns

表 熱傷深度

	症状 Symptoms	経過 Healing time	後遺症 Scarring
表皮熱傷 （Ⅰ度熱傷） Superficial (First degree burn)	発赤，浮腫 熱感・痛み Erythema, edema, hot sensation, pain	数日で治癒 Several days	傷痕は残らない None
真皮浅層および深層熱傷 （Ⅱ度熱傷） Superficial and deep dermal burn (Second degree burn)	発赤，浮腫 皮膚のはがれ 水ぶくれ 強い熱感・痛み Erythema, edema, flaky skin, blister, strong hot sensation, pain	上皮化まで2～3週間 2 to 3 weeks to epithelialization	熱傷の程度によって，傷痕が残る場合と残らない場合がある Depending on the degree of burns, scarring may occur.
皮下熱傷 （Ⅲ度熱傷） Deep burn (Third degree burn)	白色 痛みなし White skin, painless	上皮化まで2～3か月 2 to 3 months to epithelialization	傷痕が残る Scarring

●検 査 Test

■まず見て，熱傷の面積をチェックします．熱傷は，深さよりも広さが大切です．バイタルサイン（血圧，脈拍数，呼吸数など）を測定し，必要であれば検査を行います．

By visual inspection, check how large the affected area is. In burns, the extent is more important than the depth. Check vital signs. If necessary, further tests are performed.

- □血液検査　Blood test
- □エックス線検査　X-ray test
- □内視鏡（気道の熱傷が疑われる場合）　Endoscopy (When burns in the airway are suspected)

●治 療 Treatment

1．応急処置 First aid

■急いで，水で10～20分ほど冷やします．

Cool the injured area with cold water for 10 to 20 minutes.

■氷を直接当てることは避けます．

Do not put ice directly on the area.

■服は無理に脱がさず，服の上から水をかけます．冷やした後は，低体温にならないように清潔なシーツやバスタオルでくるみます．

Do not remove clothing if it is difficult. Instead, pour cold water on the top of the clothing.

■熱傷の部分は直接手で触らず，水ぶくれはつぶさないようにします．

Do not touch the injured area and do not rupture blisters.

2．局所の治療 Treatment of affected area

■傷を洗った後は，ガーゼや特殊な薬で傷をおおい，包帯やネットで固定します．

After washing the area, cover it with gauze or a specific medication and secure it with a dressing or net.

■数日間は，傷の観察を行いながら，その状況に合った薬を使います．
For days, watch the burns and use appropriate medications.

■1〜2週間たっても，傷口の皮膚ができてこない場合は，悪い組織を切り取り，皮膚の移植を考えます．
If new skin does not overlap, the additional treatment may be required such as removal of damaged tissues and grafting the skin.

3．全身の治療　Treatment to the whole body

■熱傷の範囲が広い場合（熱傷の面積が全体の 10% を超える場合）は，点滴を行い，全身の管理が必要となります．
If burns are large (larger than 10% of the body), put on a drip and treatment to the whole body are needed.

■重症の場合は，手術が必要になります．
If burns are severe, surgeries are required.

■また重症の場合は，感染や栄養の低下，潰瘍が起こることがあるので，注意が必要です．
In severe cases, infection, malnourishment, and ulcer may occur. Further care is needed.

保護者へのアドバイス　Advice to parents

★普段から，火気や高い温度のものに，子どもを近づけないようにすることが大切です．
It is important to prevent your children from close contact to fire or high heat object daily.

★冷やした後は，低体温にならないように清潔なシーツやバスタオルでくるみます．
After cooling off the area, wrap the affected area with clean sheets or bath towels to avoid hypothermia

Part 4

29 誤飲・誤嚥
Accidental ingestion, Aspiration

4. 病名を英語で説明する：英語を使った小児科診療・病名編

● こんな病気　Overview

- 誤飲とは，飲み物や食べ物でない物を，誤って飲み込んでしまうことです．
  Accidental ingestion is swallowing objects which are not food and drinks by mistake.
- 誤嚥とは，飲み物や食べ物，唾液，異物が，気管のなかに入ってしまうことです．
  Aspiration is drinks, food, saliva, and foreign objects are sucked into the airway.
- 誤飲は，1歳以下の乳児に多くみられます．
  Accidental ingestion is common in younger than 1 year of age.
- 誤嚥は，幼児に多くみられます．
  Aspiration is common in infants.

● 原　因　Cause

- 子どもに多くみられる誤飲の原因はタバコです．
  Common cause of accidental ingestion in children is tobacco.
- その他の原因に，薬や化粧品，洗剤，殺虫剤があります．
  The second common causes are medicine, cosmetics, detergents, and insecticides.
- 子どもに多くみられる誤嚥の原因は豆やおもちゃです．
  Common causes of aspiration in children are beans and toys.

● 症　状　Symptom

- 誤飲の症状は，飲み込んだ物によって異なります．
  In accidental ingestion, symptoms depend on what is swallowed.
- 誤飲では，呼吸や脈が速くなる，顔色が悪くなったりする，などの中毒症状が出ることがあります．
  Toxic symptoms may present as rapid breathing and pulse in accidental ingestion.
- 誤嚥の症状は，飲み込んだ物がどこに詰まったかによって異なります．
  Symptoms of aspiration depend on where an object is stuck.
- 誤嚥では，呼吸困難やゼーゼー，咳などの呼吸器の症状がみられます．
  In aspiration, distress in the respiratory system develops, such as difficulty in breathing, wheezing, and cough.
- 誤嚥で異物がある場所で止まると，いったん症状は消えます．
  When a foreign object is stuck at a certain place, symptoms may disappear temporarily.
- 誤嚥で異物が残っていると，発熱や咳，喀血(口から血を吐く)の症状が出てきます．
  When it does not come out, symptoms such as fever, cough, coughing up blood may develop.

● 検　査　Test

- エックス線に写る物であれば，飲み込んだ物がどこにあるのかわかりますが，エックス線

に写らない物はわかりません．

If x-ray (test) shows the object, it can be located. If it is something x-ray (test) cannot detect, not be used to locate the object.

- □エックス線検査　X-ray (test)
- □CT 検査　CT scan
- □MRI 検査　MRI
- □肺血流シンチグラフィー　Lung perfusion scintigraphy
- □気管支鏡・気管支ファイバースコープ　Bronchoscope, bronchofiberscope

●治　療　Treatment
【誤飲の治療　Treatment for accidental ingestion】

1．異物の確認　Confirm the foreign object
- ■まず，本当に飲んだのか，何をどれくらい飲んだのか，症状はないかなどの確認をします．
Check if it is swallowed, what and how much is swallowed, and there are any symptoms.

2．吐かせてよい物かどうかの判断　Determine if it is safe to induce vomiting
- ■誤飲したものの中には，吐かせてよいものといけないものがあります．
Some swallowed items are not safe to spit out.
- ■強酸性・強アルカリ性の物や，石油製品，先の尖ったものなどは，吐かせてはいけません．
If swallowed ones are strong acidic and alkaline objects, petroleum products, and sharp objects, do not let your children spit it out.

3．吐かせ方　How to induce vomiting
- ■誤飲の場合は，スプーンを舌の奥にあて，下に押して吐かせます．
In case of accidental ingestion, press a spoon on the tongue deep in the mouth and let your children vomit.
- ■吐かせた後は，左を下にして寝かせ，胃の内容物が腸に流れていかないようにします．
After making them vomit, lay them down on the left side, and prevent the contents of the stomach drain into the intestine.
- ■誤嚥の場合は，背中を勢いよく叩きます．体が大きい子には，背中から手をまわし，こぶしで胃を突きあげます（図）．
In case aspiration, slap their back with force. When your children are big enough, support their back with your hand, and push up their stomach with your fist (Heimlich maneuver).

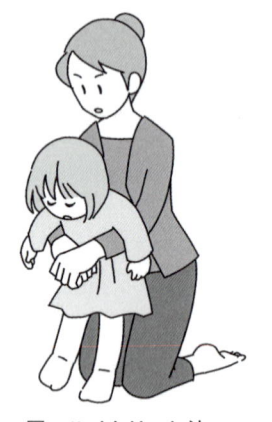

図　ハイムリッヒ法
Heimlich maneuver

4．胃洗浄　Gastric irrigation
- ■誤飲して，1時間以内であれば，病院で胃のなかを洗う処置を行うことがあります．
Within an hour after swallowing a foreign object, procedure to washout the stomach may be administered at hospitals.

5．異物の摘出　Removal of a foreign object
- ■異物が気道にある場合は，のどの奥をのぞく道具を使って，直接取り出します．
If a foreign object is stuck in the airway, remove it directly by using a nasopharyngo scope.

29. 誤飲・誤嚥　Accidental ingestion, Aspiration

【誤嚥の治療　Treatment for aspiration】

1. 異物の摘出　Removal of a foreign object
   - 異物が気管にある場合は，気管支鏡や気管支ファイバースコープを使って，取り出します．
   If an object is stuck in the airway, remove it with a bronchoscope or bronchofiberscope.

2. 手術
   - 気管支鏡や気管支ファイバースコープで取り出すことができない場合は，手術が必要になります．
   If a bronchoscope or bronchofiberscope cannot remove it, surgical removal is needed.

●治療の合併症　Complication

1. 誤嚥の危険　Complication of aspiration
   - 意識障害がある状態で胃洗浄を行った場合，誤嚥の危険があります．
   When disturbance of consciousness is present, gastric irrigation may cause aspiration.

2. 出血や穿孔の危険　Risks of bleeding and perforation
   - 胃洗浄や，気管支鏡・気管支ファイバースコープでは，食道や胃，気道，気管支の損傷を起こす危険があります．
   Gastric irrigation, bronchoscope, and bronchofiberscope have risks causing damage to the esophagus, stomach, airway, and bronchi.

3. 麻酔　Anesthesia
   - 気管支鏡や気管支ファイバースコープを行う場合，全身麻酔が必要になる事があります．
   Procedures with bronchoscope and bronchofiberscope may require general anesthesia.

保護者へのアドバイス　Advice to parents

★子どもが誤飲した場合，誤飲したものの残りや，空のビン，メーカーの説明書などを持って，病院を受診しましょう．
When your children swallow something by mistake, bring what is left, or empty bottle, or manufacture's instruction with you.

★タバコなど，誤飲しやすいものを，子どもの周りに置かないようにしましょう．
Keep objects easy to swallow such as tobacco away from your children's reach.

★液体に溶けたタバコは中毒を起こすことがあり，ジュースなどの空き缶を灰皿がわりにしないようにしましょう．
Tobacco dissolved in water may cause poisoning. Do not use empty juice cans as ash trays.

★吐かせてはいけない強酸性・強アルカリ性のものとして，トイレの洗剤やカビ取り洗剤などがあります．
For strong acid・alkaline products you must not have your children vomit. These are bathroom cleaners and mold removers.

5章

診断書・証明書編
Medical certificate・prescription

The aim of this chapter

　日本でよく利用される各種証明書とその英語版を並べて紹介. とくに予防接種証明書は重要な書類ですので, 記入例や注意点を詳しく紹介しました.
　また, 予防接種証明書, 健康診断書, 診断書は診断と治療社HP (http://www.shindan.co.jp/) より英語版フォームをダウンロードすることができます.
※144ページ以降は176％でコピーすると, およそA4サイズになります.

●証明書テンプレートのダウンロードサービスについて

　各種証明書の中でも，使用頻度の高い「予防接種証明書」「健康診断書」「診断書」の3点の英語版をテンプレートとして，使用できるようにしました．データは，診断と治療社のHPより，以下の方法にてダウンロードできます．記入方法，日本語訳などは本書を参照ください．
　2）健康診断書と3）診断書の選択記入式の箇所は，印刷後手書で丸をつけるか，片方を消して下さい．

1）予防接種証明書

```
CERTIFICATE OF PREVIOUS VACCINATION AND RECORDS OF DISEASES

                                                    Date:

Name:              Date of birth:          Gender:

1) Records of Vaccination
  | Type of Vaccination | Date |

2) Results of Serum Antibody Titer
  | Name of Disease | Date of Sampling | Antibody Titer | Determination |

This is to certify that these data come from our medical investigations and records.
```

ダウンロード方法

① 診断と治療社HP（http://www.shindan.co.jp/）へアクセスして，書籍名を入力．
② 書籍詳細ページの［証明書のテンプレートへ］をクリックしてください．
③ ダウンロードページがあらわれますので，そこからダウンロードしてご使用ください．
※テンプレートはPDF形式です
※使用には，Adobe®Reader®8以上が必要となります
※ダウンロード後，記入箇所に入力して保存・印刷が可能ですが，各欄によって字数に限りがあります

証明書テンプレートのダウンロードサービスについて

2）健康診断書

Physical Examination

Name		Blood Type	(A・B・AB・O), RhD (＋・－)
Sex	(M　F)	Red Blood Count (10000/μL)	
Date of Birth		Hemoglobin (g/dL)	
Age	(　Years　　Months)	Hematocrit (%)	
Medical History		White Blood Cells Count (/μL)	
Allergy		Neutrophil Rate (%)	
Allergy to Medication		Eosinophil Rate (%)	
Allergy to Food		Basophil Rate (%)	
Height (cm)		Monocyte Rate (%)	
Weight (kg)		Lymphocyte Rate (%)	
Head Circumference (cm)		Platelet (10000/μL)	
Systolic BP (mmHg)		Total Protein (g/dL)	
Diastolic BP (mmHg)		Albumi (g/dL)	
Pulse (time/min)		Total Bilirubin (mg/dL)	
Vision (Left/Right)	[　　・　　]	AST (IU/L)	
Corrected Vision (L/R)	[　　・　　]	ALT (IU/L)	
Color Vision	(Normal・Abnormal)	LDH (IU/L)	
Hearing (Left)	1000Hz　　dB(Normal・Abnormal)	Cholinesterase (mg/dL)	
The Same as Above	4000Hz　　dB(Normal・Abnormal)	Total Cholesterol (mg/dL)	
Hearing (Right)	1000Hz　　dB(Normal・Abnormal)	Newtral Fat (mg/dL)	
The Same as Above	4000Hz　　dB(Normal・Abnormal)	Urea Nitrogen (mg/dL)	
Physical Examination		Creatinine (mg/dL)	
Chest X-ray		Uric Acid (mg/dL)	
EKG		Fasting Blood Glucose Level (mg/dL)	
Urinary Protein	(Negative・Positive)	HBs Antigen	
Urinary Sugar	(Negative・Positive)	HBsAntibody	
Occult Blood in Urine	(Negative・Positive)	HCV Antibody	
Urinary Sediment	(Normal・Abnormal)	HIV Screening	
Others		Overall Health Condition	

The above stated patient is under my care.

Date

Physician's Printed Name and Signature

Name/Address

Tel/Fax/E-mail

3）診断書

Medical Examination Report

Name :

Date of Birth :

Sex: (Male・Female)

For the patient stated above:

Diagnosis:

Remarks:

Date_____

Physician's signature_____

Physician's printed name_____

Hospital's Name and Department_____

Address_____

Tel/Fax/Email Address_____

●予防接種証明書／フォーム

Kawasaki Hospital
Kawasaki Medical School
2-1-80, Nakasange, Kita-ku, Okayama, 700-8505, Japan
Tel: +81-86-225-2111, Fax: +81-86-232-8343

CERTIFICATE OF PREVIOUS VACCINATION AND RECORDS OF DISEASES
予防接種と既往疾患，血清抗体価に関する証明書

❶ (レターヘッド)

Date: ❷　日付

Name: ❸　氏名
Date of birth: ❹　生年月日
Gender: 性別

1) Records of Vaccination　予防接種歴

Type of Vaccination 種類	Date 接種日 ❹

2) Records of Past History　既往疾患

Name of Disease 疾患名	Date 罹患日 ❹

2) Results of Serum Antibody Titer　血清抗体価

Name of Disease 疾患名	Date of Sampling ❹ 採血日	Antibody Titer 抗体価	Determination 測定法

This is to certify that these data come from our medical investigations and records.
上記の記載は，診療録，問診，検査結果の記録などに基づいたものであることを証明する．

❺
Takashi Nakano, M.D.

❻ Department of Pediatrics, Kawasaki Hospital, Kawasaki Medical School
2-1-80, Nakasange, Kita-ku, Okayama, 700-8505, Japan
Tel: +81-86-225-2111, Fax: +81-86-232-8343
e-mail: pediatr@med.kawasaki-m.ac.jp

❼

---

❶ 医療機関のレターヘッドがある用紙を使うのが望ましい．

❷ 書類を発行した日はかならず記載する．アメリカは＜月／日／年＞，その他の国は＜日／月／年＞の順に記載することが一般的．

❸ 姓名の記載は，ローマ字綴りにしパスポート記載と同一にすることが望ましい．

❹ 生年月日や接種日などの日付は西暦で記載する．アメリカは＜月／日／年＞，その他の国は＜日／月／年＞の順に記載することが一般的．

❺ 医師名の印字とともに，かならず署名をする．

❻ 医療機関名，診療科，所在地，電話番号，FAX，e-mail などを記載する．

❼ 押印の習慣がない国も多いが，英文の病院印はあるとよい．

●予防接種証明書／記入例①

```
                    Kawasaki Hospital
                    Kawasaki Medical School

              2-1-80, Nakasange, Kita-ku, Okayama, 700-8505, Japan
              Tel: +81-86-225-2111,  Fax: +81-86-232-8343
         CERTIFICATE OF PREVIOUS VACCINATION AND RECORDS OF DISEASES

                                              Date:  April 8, 2011

 Name:                Date of birth: January 14, 2007   Gender:  Female

 1) Records of Vaccination
```

Type of Vaccination		Date
DaPT[1)]	1st ❶	April 20, 2007
DaPT	2nd	May 18, 2007
DaPT	3rd	June 15, 2007
TOPV[2)]	1st ❶	June 22, 2007
TOPV	2nd	October 23, 2007
MR[3)] ❶		January 15, 2008
Varicella		February 19, 2008
Mumps		February 19, 2008
JE[4)]	1st	March 24, 2010
JE	2nd	April 21, 2010

❶ 1) DaPT: diphtheria, acellular pertussis, tetanus combined vaccine
2) TOPV: trivalent live attenuated oral polio vaccine
3) MR: measles, rubella combined vaccine   4) JE: japanese encephalitis vaccine

2) Results of Serum Antibody Titer

Name of Disease	Date of Sampling ❷	Antibody Titer ❷	Determination ❷
Measles	March 3, 2011	1 : 512, poisitive ❸	PA ❹
Rubella	March 3, 2011	less than 1 : 8, negative ❸	HI ❹
Mumps	March 3, 2011	23.5 EU(EIA Unit), positive ❸	EIA-IgG ❹
Varicella	March 3, 2011	1 : 32, positive ❸	IAHA ❹

This is to certify that these data come from our medical investigations and records.

                                        Takashi Nakano, M.D.

       Department of Pediatrics, Kawasaki Hospital, Kawasaki Medical School
              2-1-80, Nakasange, Kita-ku, Okayama, 700-8505, Japan
              Tel: +81-86-225-2111, Fax: +81-86-232-8343
                         e-mail: pediatr@med.kawasaki-m.ac.jp

---

❶ ワクチンや疾患名は出来る限り略称にしない方が望ましいが，略す場合には脚注を付す．
例：DaPT（ジフテリア・無細胞型百日咳・破傷風混合ワクチン），DT（ジフテリア・破傷風混合ワクチン）TOPV（3価弱毒化経口生ポリオワクチン），IPV（不活化ポリオワクチン），MR（麻疹・風疹混合ワクチン），MMR（麻疹・ムンプス・風疹混合ワクチン），JE（日本脳炎ワクチン）

❷ 血清抗体価については，抗体価のみならず，測定日，測定に用いた方法も記載する．

❸ 抗体価について，測定値「512倍」は「1：512」と記載する．「8倍未満」は「less than 1：8」となる．測定方法が酵素免疫法（enzyme immunoassay, EIA）の場合は，絶対値（EIA単位）を記載する．結果の解釈（陽性，陰性）も併せて記載する．

❹ 抗体測定に用いた方法を記載する．
例：赤血球凝集抑制法（hemagglutination inhibition, HI），中和法（neutralization test, NT），酵素免疫法（enzyme immunoassay, EIA；IgG抗体やIgM抗体など免疫グロブリン分画別の抗体価が測定できる），粒子凝集法（particle agglutination, PA），免疫粘着血球凝集反応（immune adherence hemagglutination, IAHA），化学発光免疫測定法（chemiluminescent immunoassay, CLIA）など

●予防接種証明書／記入例②

Kawasaki Hospital
Kawasaki Medical School

2-1-80, Nakasange, Kita-ku, Okayama, 700-8505, Japan
Tel: +81-86-225-2111, Fax: +81-86-232-8343

CERTIFICATE OF PREVIOUS VACCINATION AND RECORDS OF DISEASES

Date: April 8, 2011

Name: _____   Date of birth: June 21, 1990   Gender: Male

1) Records of Vaccination

Type of Vaccination	Date
DaPT[1]	December 24, 1990
BCG 1st	February 15, 1991
BCG 2nd	May 15, 1997
Hepatitis B 1st	February 14, 2011
Hepatitis B 2nd	March 14, 2011

1) DaPT: diphtheria, acellular pertussis, tetanus combined vaccine

2) Records of Past History

Name of Disease	Date
Measles	July, 1993
Varicella	April, 1994
Mumps	around 5 years old
Rubella	during junior high school days

* He developed an anaphylactic reaction 10 hours after receiving a DaPT vaccine in December, 1990. Although definitive causal relationship between the reaction and the vaccine is not clarified, subsequent DaPT vaccinations were omitted to minimize the risk of a similar adverse reaction. ❶

* He received a BCG vaccination at the age of 7 months and 6 years as routine vaccination for all children in Japan. Now he has tested positive in a tuberculin test (positive conversion by the BCG vaccination) at 20 years old. He doesn't have any clinical evidence of tuberculosis on physical examination, and his chest X-ray reveals no abnormality. ❷

This is to certify that these data come from our medical investigations and records.

Takashi Nakano, M.D.

Department of Pediatrics, Kawasaki Hospital, Kawasaki Medical School
2-1-80, Nakasange, Kita-ku, Okayama, 700-8505, Japan
Tel: +81-86-225-2111, Fax: +81-86-232-8343
e-mail: pediatr@med.kawasaki-m.ac.jp

【例文として挙げた特記事項❶, ❷の日本語訳】

❶（規定回数の DaPT 接種が行われていない理由の説明）
彼は，1990 年 12 月に DaPT ワクチンを接種した 10 時間後にアナフィラキシー反応を呈した既往がある．DaPT ワクチンが本反応の原因であったかどうかの因果関係は明らかでないが，同様の副反応発現の危険性を出来る限り避けるために，その後の DaPT 追加接種は行わなかった．

❷（BCG がすべての子どもたちを対象に実施されているわが国の定期接種制度の説明；ツベルクリン反応検査が陽性の場合，BCG 接種を行ってない国では結核感染と混同されることがあるので，その点も記載すると有用である．）
彼は生後 7 か月時と 6 歳時に，日本ではすべての子どもたちを対象として実施される定期接種として BCG を接種した．20 歳となった現在，ツベルクリン反応検査の判定は陽性，BCG 接種による陽転である．診察所見に結核を疑わせる徴候はなく，胸部エックス線検査も正常である．

【❶，❷以外の例文を日英文対比で下記に示します】

【日本文】彼女は食物アレルギーがあり，卵を摂取すると血圧低下，呼吸困難などのアナフィラキシー様反応を起こす．
　ニワトリ胚細胞の組織培養で製造される麻疹ワクチンには卵成分と交差反応を示す蛋白はほとんど含まれないが，本児が麻疹ワクチン接種により同様の反応を来たす可能性を完全に否定はできない．
　したがって，麻疹ワクチンは接種しなかった．

【英文】Ingestion of egg causes severe anaphylactic reactions such as drops in blood pressure and respiratory difficulty because of her food allergy.
　Though the measles vaccine produced by tissue culture of chicken embryo cell contains almost no proteins cross-reactive with egg ingredients, we are not completely sure whether the vaccine induce similar reaction or not.
　Therefore, we have not vaccinated her against measles.

【日本文】日本では2002年まで小中学生のツベルクリン反応陰性者に対してBCG接種が行われていた．
　2011年3月8日に彼女に実施したツベルクリン反応の判定結果は陽性（硬結の長径18 mm）だが，これは過去のBCG接種による細胞性免疫の感作を意味するものである．

【英文】BCG had been administered to students with negative results of tuberculin test in primary school and junior high school until 2002 in Japan.
　She tested positive in the tuberculin test(major axis of induration with 18 mm)on March 8, 2011, hence her former BCG vaccination was concluded to sensitize her to cellular immunity.

●健康診断書／様式（日本語，英語）　英語版フォーマットはダウンロード可

健康診断書

氏名		血液型	(A・B・AB・O), RhD (＋・－)
性別	（ 男 ・ 女 ）	赤血球数(万/μL)	
生年月日		血色素量(g/dL)	
年齢	（　　歳　　か月）	ヘマトクリット(%)	
既往歴		白血球数(/μL)	
アレルギー歴		好中球比率(%)	
投与禁の薬剤		好酸球比率(%)	
禁止飲食物		好塩基球比率(%)	
身長(cm)		単球比率(%)	
体重(kg)		リンパ球比率(%)	
頭囲(cm)		血小板数(万/μL)	
最高血圧(mmHg)		総蛋白(g/dL)	
最低血圧(mmHg)		アルブミン(g/dL)	
脈拍(回/分)		総ビリルビン(mg/dL)	
視力〔左・右〕	[　　・　　]	AST (IU/L)	
矯正視力〔左・右〕	[　　・　　]	ALT (IU/L)	
色神	（ 正常 ・ 異常 ）	LDH (IU/L)	
聴力〔左〕	1000Hz　dB (正常・異常)	コリンエステラーゼ(mg/dL)	
同上	4000Hz　dB (正常・異常)	総コレステロール(mg/dL)	
聴力〔右〕	1000Hz　dB (正常・異常)	中性脂肪(mg/dL)	
同上	4000Hz　dB (正常・異常)	尿素窒素(mg/dL)	
身体の理学的所見		クレアチニン(mg/dL)	
胸部X線所見		尿酸(mg/dL)	
心電図所見		空腹時血糖(mg/dL)	
尿蛋白	（ 陰性 ・ 陽性 ）	HBs抗原	
尿糖	（ 陰性 ・ 陽性 ）	HBs抗体	
尿潜血	（ 陰性 ・ 陽性 ）	HCV抗体	
尿沈渣	（ 正常 ・ 異常 ）	HIV検査	
その他の特記事項		総合判定	

上記の通り診断する

　　　年　　月　　日

医師氏名（印字・署名）

医療機関名と所在地

電話・Fax・メールなど

Physical Examination

Name		Blood Type	(A・B・AB・O), RhD (＋・－)
Sex	(M　F)	Red Blood Count (10000/μL)	
Date of Birth		Hemoglobin (g/dL)	
Age	(　Years　Months)	Hematocrit (%)	
Medical History		White Blood Cells Count (/μL)	
Allergy		Neutrophil Rate (%)	
Allergy to Medication		Eosinophil Rate (%)	
Allergy to Food		Basophil Rate (%)	
Height (cm)		Monocyte Rate (%)	
Weight (kg)		Lymphocyte Rate (%)	
Head Circumference (cm)		Platelet (10000/μL)	
Systolic BP (mmHg)		Total Protein (g/dL)	
Diastolic BP (mmHg)		Albumi (g/dL)	
Pulse (time/min)		Total Bilirubin (mg/dL)	
Vision (Left/Right)	[　　・　　]	AST (IU/L)	
Corrected Vision (L/R)	[　　・　　]	ALT (IU/L)	
Color Vision	(Normal・Abnormal)	LDH (IU/L)	
Hearing (Left)	1000Hz　dB (Normal・Abnormal)	Cholinesterase (mg/dL)	
The Same as Above	4000Hz　dB (Normal・Abnormal)	Total Cholesterol (mg/dL)	
Hearing (Right)	1000Hz　dB (Normal・Abnormal)	Newtral Fat (mg/dL)	
The Same as Above	4000Hz　dB (Normal・Abnormal)	Urea Nitrogen (mg/dL)	
Physical Examination		Creatinine (mg/dL)	
Chest X-ray		Uric Acid (mg/dL)	
EKG		Fasting Blood Glucose Level (mg/dL)	
Urinary Protein	(Negative・Positive)	HBs Antigen	
Urinary Sugar	(Negative・Positive)	HBsAntibody	
Occult Blood in Urine	(Negative・Positive)	HCV Antibody	
Urinary Sediment	(Normal・Abnormal)	HIV Screening	
Others		Overall Health Condition	

The above stated patient is under my care.

Date

Physician's Printed Name and Signature

Name/Address

Tel/Fax/E-mail

健康診断書，診断書

● 診断書／様式（日本語，英語）　英語版フォーマットはダウンロード可

Medical Examination Report

Name :

Date of Birth :

Sex: (Male ・ Female)

For the patient stated above :

Diagnosis :

Remarks :

Date _____

Physician's signature _____

Physician's printed name _____

Hospital's Name and Department _____

Address _____

Tel/Fax/Email Address _____

診断書

氏名：

生年月日：

性別：(男性 ・ 女性)

上記の者について，以下のように診断する。

病名：

付記事項：

　年　　月　　日

医師氏名（署名）_____

医師氏名（印字）_____

医療機関および診療科名 _____

医療機関住所 _____

電話，Fax，メールアドレス　など

●説明と同意書／様式（日本語）

説明場所：

説明日時： 年　月　日　時　分から　時　分まで

説明医師氏名（印字と署名）：

立会人（印字と署名）：

――――――――――――――――――――――

上記の通り説明を受け、理解し同意した。

同意年月日： 年　月　日

患者氏名（印字と署名）：

患者代理人氏名（印字と署名）：

患者代理人の続柄：《父・母・その他親族や関係者（　　）》

代理人署名の事由：《児が低年齢・両親などが連絡不能・その他（　　）》

立会人（印字と署名）：

説明と同意の記録

患者氏名：

生年月日：

性別：（男性 ・ 女性 ）

本患者について、以下のように説明と同意を行った。

説明と同意事項：　　　　　　　　　　に関する説明と同意

医師・コメディカルからの説明内容：

患者・患者家族や関係者からの質問：

質問に対する医師・コメディカルからの回答：

――――――――――――――――――――――

上記の通り説明した。

146

●説明と同意書／様式（英語）

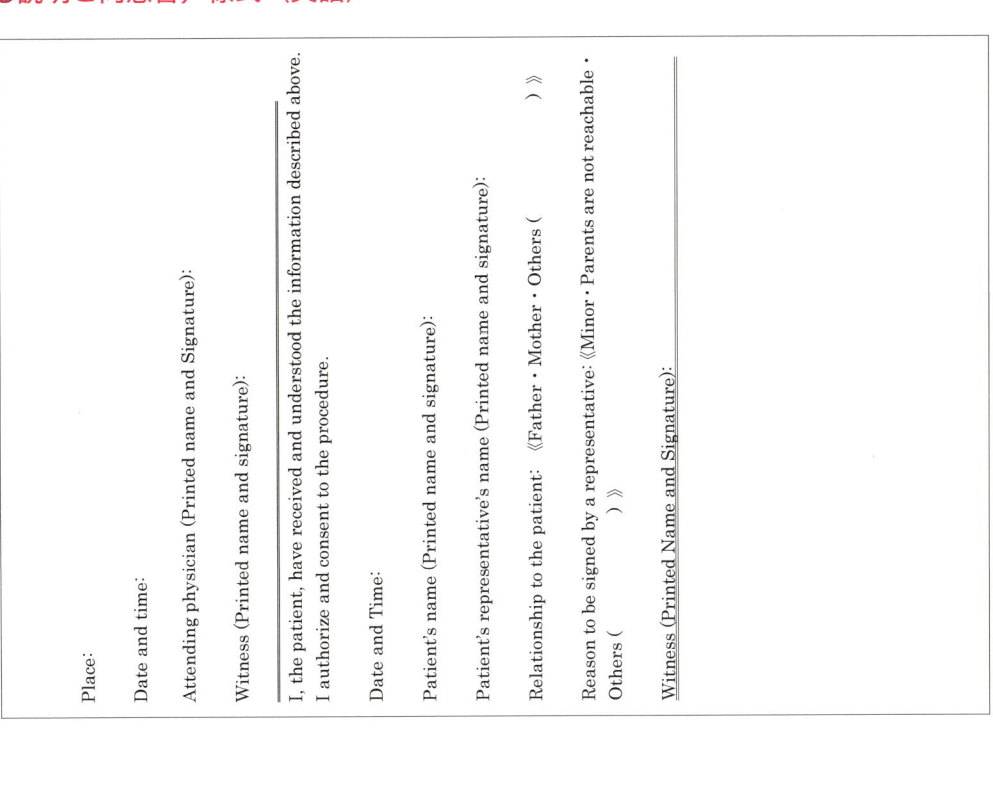

Place:

Date and time:

Attending physician (Printed name and signature):

Witness (Printed name and signature):

I, the patient, have received and understood the information described above. I authorize and consent to the procedure.

Date and Time:

Patient's name (Printed name and signature):

Patient's representative's name (Printed name and signature):

Relationship to the patient: 《Father・Mother・Others (　　　)》

Reason to be signed by a representative: 《Minor・Parents are not reachable・Others (　　　)》

Witness (Printed Name and Signature):

Informed Consent Form

Patient's Name:

Date of Birth:

Sex: (Male　　Female):

The above stated patient has received the following information and given his/her consent to the operation or procedure recommended to him/her. Information and the performance of the operation or procedure authorized and consented by the patient regarding _____

Doctors・medical team have explained:

Patient・family members・responsible party have asked:

Doctors・medical team have answered:

I, the undersigned physician, certify that I have discussed the procedure described above with the patient (and or the patient's representative).

●通院証明書／様式（日本語，英語）

Outpatient Visits

Name:

Date of Birth:

Sex: (Male ・ Female)

This is to certify that the above stated person was under my care as an outpatient.

Diagnosis:

Duration:

From _____ to _____, this patient had _____ visits.

Date:

Physician's signature _____

Physician's printed name _____

Hospital's Name and Department _____

Address _____

Tel/Fax/Email Address _____

通院証明書

氏名：

生年月日：

性別：(男性 ・ 女性)

上記の者、以下のように当医療機関に通院したことを証明する。

病名：

通院期間：　年　月　日から　年　月　日までの期間のうち、
　　　　　　日間通院

　年　月　日

医師氏名（署名）：

医師氏名（印字）：

医療機関および診療科名：

医療機関住所：

電話，Fax，メールアドレス など：

通院証明書，入院証明書

●入院証明書／様式（日本語，英語）

Duration of Inpatient Stay

Name:

Date of Birth

Sex: (Male・Female)

This is to certify that the above stated person was under my care as an inpatient.

Diagnosis

Duration

From _____ to _____, _____ days

Date

Physician's signature _____

Physician's printed name _____

Hospital's Name and Department _____

Address _____

Tel/Fax/Email Address _____

入院証明書

氏名：

生年月日：

性別：（男性 ・ 女性 ）

上記の者，以下のように当医療機関に入院したことを証明する。

病名：

入院期間：　　年　　月　　日から　　年　　月　　日まで　　日間

　　　　年　　月　　日

医師氏名（署名）：

医師氏名（印字）：

医療機関および診療科名：

医療機関住所：

電話，Fax，メールアドレス　など：

●入院診療計画書(例1)／記入例(日本語,英語)

Inpatient Diagnosis and Treatment Plan Form (Sample 1)

Patient's Name: _____
Date of Birth: _____
Sex: (Male ・ Female)   Date _____

Department・Room	West Wing Inpatient Unit 3rd Floor・Room 311
Diagnosis	Bacterial pneumonia, Dehydration
Other possible diagnosis	Viral pneumonia, watch out for complications from bronchial asthma such as respiratory insufficiency and cardiac failure.
Symptoms	Fever, cough, stridor, dyspnea, loss of appetite, oliguria
Treatment plan	・Intravenous infusion, instillation of antibacterial drug ・If necessary, oxygen is administered.
Tests and testing schedule	・Blood test, urine test, chest x-ray ・If necessary, blood test and chest x-ray are performed multiple times. ・Periodic observation of oxygen saturation as measured using pulse oximetry (SpO_2)
Surgical procedure and date of the surgery	There is no surgery scheduled.
Estimated duration of inpatient stay	About 1 week
Others (Care, rehabilitation plan)	・Appropriate infusion management, inspection and maintenance of the medical equipment in the patient's room ・Make the best effort to provide the patient with rest, appropriate nourishment, and hygiene.

Note 1) Current diagnosis may change by further testing results.
Note 2) Duration of inpatient stay is estimated by the current condition.
Physician's name (Printed name and signature) _____

Nurse or other medical provider's name(Printed name and signature)
_____

Patient's Signature _____

Patient's family or responsible party's signature _____

Relationship to the patient _____

入院診療計画書(例1)

患者氏名：
生年月日：
性別：(男性 ・ 女性)   年　月　日

病棟・病室	3階西病棟・311室
病名	細菌性肺炎,脱水症
他に考えられる病名	・ウイルス性肺炎,呼吸不全,心不全など ・気管支喘息の合併がないか注意します
症状	発熱,咳,喘鳴,呼吸困難,食欲不振,尿量減少
治療計画	・経静脈輸液,抗菌薬の点滴静注 ・必要があれば酸素投与を行います
検査内容および日程	・血液検査,尿検査,胸部X線検査 ・必要に応じて,複数回数の血液検査や胸部X線検査を行います ・経皮的血液酸素飽和度(SpO_2)の定期的観察
手術内容及び日程	今のところ,手術予定はありません
推定される入院期間	約1週間程度
その他 (看護,リハビリテーション等の計画)	・適切な輸液管理,入院環境の整備 ・安静,適切な栄養,身体の清潔保持に努めます

注1) 病名等は現時点で考えられるものであり,今後検査を進めるにしたがって変わり得るものである。
注2) 入院期間については,現時点で予想されるものである。

医師氏名 (印字と署名)：

看護師など氏名 (印字と署名)：

　　　　　　　　　　　　　　患者名：

　　　患者家族,関係者署名：

150

入院診療計画書

●入院診療計画書（例2）／記入例（日本語，英語）

Inpatient Diagnosis and Treatment Plan Form (Sample 2)

Patient's Name: _____
Date of Birth: _____
Sex: (Male・Female)

Date _____

Department・Room	・Intensive Care Unit
Diagnosis	Status epilepticus
Other possible diagnosis	・Any disease associated with repeated seizures ・Differential diagnosis is made such as influenza encephalopathy and epilepsy, etc.
Symptoms	Fever, convulsion, disturbance of consciousness, and respiratory arrest
Treatment plan	・Intensive care with ventilator. ・Treatment is based on the moment by moment condition.
Tests and testing schedule	・Head CT scan, EEG, blood test, urine test ・Other tests may be performed depending on the condition. ・Tests are done to manage the respiratory and circulatory system.
Surgical procedure and date of the surgery	Depending on the condition. We will inform you when it becomes necessary.
Estimated duration of inpatient stay	About 3 weeks
Others (Care, rehabilitation plan)	・Intensive care management ・Rehabilitation might be planned to recover bodily function.

Note 1) Current diagnosis may change by further testing results.
Note 2) Duration of inpatient stay is estimated by the current condition.

Physician's name (Printed name and signature): _____

Nurse or other medical provider's name (Printed name and Signature) _____

Patient's Signature _____

Patient's family or responsible party's signature _____

Relationship to the patient _____

入院診療計画書（例2）

患者氏名：
生年月日：　　　年　　月　　日
性別：（男性　・　女性）

　　　　　棟

病・病室	集中治療室
病名	けいれん重積
他に考えられる病名	・けいれん発作が反復する各種疾患 ・インフルエンザ脳症、てんかんなどを鑑別診断します
症状	発熱、けいれん発作、意識障害、呼吸停止
治療計画	・人口呼吸管理など集中治療を行います ・時々刻々の病状に応じて対処します
検査内容および日程	・頭部CT検査、脳波検査、血液検査、尿検査など ・その他必要に応じて、各種検査を実施します ・呼吸・循環管理などに実施な検査を行います
手術内容及び日程	病状に応じて実施の必要性がでてきたら説明します
推定される入院期間	約3週間程度
その他（看護、リハビリテーション等の計画）	・全身の集中管理に必要な看護や管理を行います ・一定期間経過後に、身体機能回復のためのリハビリテーションを計画する可能性があります

注1）病名等は現時点で考えられるものであり、今後精査を進めるにしたがって変わり得るものである。
注2）入院期間については、現時点で予想されるものである。

医師氏名（印字と署名）：_____

看護師など氏名（印字と署名）：_____

患者署名：_____

患者家族、関係者署名：_____

●通園・登校許可書／様式（日本語，英語）

Return to School

Name:

Date of Birth

Sex: (Male・Female)

The above stated person has been under my care and is able to return to school.

Diagnosis:

Sick leave-
from _____ to _____

Date

Physician's signature _____

Physician's printed name _____

Hospital's Name and Department _____

Address _____

Tel/Fax/Email Address _____

通園・登校許可書

氏名：

生年月日：

性別：（男性 ・ 女性 ）

病名：

上記の者，以下のように療養中であったが，このたび軽快し通園・登校が可能であると判断する。

通園・登校停止期間：
　年　月　日から　年　月　日まで

　年　月　日

医師氏名（署名）：

医師氏名（印字）：

医療機関および診療科名：

医療機関住所：

電話，Fax，メールアドレス など：

●分娩予定日証明書／様式（日本語，英語）

Expected Date of Delivery

Name: _____

Date of Birth _____

This is to certify that the above stated person's expected date of delivery is
_____

Date _____

                       Physician's signature _____

                       Physician's printed name _____

                       Hospital's Name and Department _____

                       Address _____

                       Tel/Fax/Email Address _____

分娩予定日証明書

氏名：

生年月日：

上記の者，分娩予定日は　　年　　月　　日であると証明する。

　　　　　年　　月　　日

                       医師氏名（署名）：

                       医師氏名（印字）：

                       医療機関および診療科名：

                       医療機関住所：

                       電話，Fax，メールアドレス　など：

●分娩証明書／様式（日本語，英語）

Labor and Delivery Certificate

Name

Date of Birth

Sex: Female

This is to certify that the above stated person gave a birth as follows:

Delivered Date: _____ Time _____

Child's Sex: (Boy ・ Girl)

Birth Weight _____ g

Gestational age _____ weeks ____ days

Date _____

　　　　　　　　　　　　　　Physician's signature _____

　　　　　　　　　　　　　　Physician's printed name _____

　　　　　　　　　　　　　　Hospital's Name and Department _____

　　　　　　　　　　　　　　Address _____

　　　　　　　　　　　　　　Tel/Fax/Email Address _____

分娩証明書

氏名：

生年月日：

性別：女性

上記の者について，以下のように証明する。

分娩日時： 年　月　日　時　分

出生児の性別：(男児・女児)

出生児の体重：　　　グラム

出生児の在胎週数：　　週

年　月　日

　　　　　　　　　　　　医師氏名（署名）：

　　　　　　　　　　　　医師氏名（印字）：

　　　　　　　　　　　　医療機関および診療科名：

　　　　　　　　　　　　医療機関住所：

　　　　　　　　　　　　電話, Fax, メールアドレス　など：

索引

数

1 か月健診　57
1 歳 6 か月健診　59
1 歳健診　59
3〜4 か月健診　58
3 歳健診　60
4 歳健診　61
5 歳健診　61
6〜7 か月健診　58
9〜10 か月健診　59

欧文

accidental ingestion　133
acute otitis medeia　76
aspiration　133
atopic dermatits　112
A 型肝炎　56
BCG　55
bronchial asthma　109
burns　130
B 型肝炎　56
certificate of previous vaccination and records of diseases　140, 141, 142
chicken pox　98
common cold　68
congenital heart disease　106
contusion　127
diabetes mellitus　121
DPT　55
duration of inpatient stay　149
epidemic parotitis　96
epliepsy　104
exantema subitum　84
expected date of delivery　151
febrile seizures　86
food allergies　115
food poisoning and food contamination　80
gastroenteritis　78
gloup A streptococcal infections　72
hand-foot-and mouth disease　88
herpangina　90
hives　118
influenza　70
informed consent form　147
inpatient diagnosis and treatment plan form　150, 151
kawasaki disease　102
labor and delivery certificate　154
measles　92
medical examination report　145
MMR　56
MR　55
mumps　96
obesity　124

otafuku-cold　96
outpatient visits　148
pertussis　100
physical examination　144
pneumonia　74
return to school　152
roseola infantum　84
rubella　94
trauma　127
urinariy tract infection（UTI）　82
urticaria　118
varicella　98
wooping cough　100

和文

あ

あいさつ　10
悪性　31
アトピー性皮膚炎　55, 112
アレルギー　19
アレルゲン　31
育成医療　5
痛みの程度　14
胃粘膜保護薬　36
医療費　5
医療保険　11, 12, 47
院外処方せん　47
インシュリン　20
インフォームド・コンセント　4
インフルエンザ　56, 70

うえお

うがい薬　36
エックス線検査　27
嘔吐　54, 65
悪寒　16
おたふくかぜ　55, 96
おねしょ　65

か

海外旅行保険　10
外国語版母子健康手帳　4
外国人家族　2
外国人登録　5
外国人の子ども　2
外傷　127
喀痰検査　27
カ氏　14, 17
かぜ症候群　68
カプセル　44
花粉アレルギー　21
かゆみ止め　36
ガラクトース血症　64

155

顆粒　44
川崎病　102
ガン　20
肝炎　31
緩下薬　36
肝機能　20
完全看護　33
還付　49

き
既往歴　19
気管支拡張薬　36
気管支ぜんそく　55, 109
機嫌　54
急性胃腸炎　78
急性糸球体腎炎　72, 73
急性中耳炎　76
吸入薬　36, 40
去痰薬　36

くけ
空腹時　35
　―血糖値　31
クレジットカード　47
激痛　16
血圧　27
血圧降下薬　36
血液検査　27
血管拡張薬　36
血栓溶解薬　36
血便　16
解熱薬　35, 36
下痢　14, 16, 17, 54, 65
下痢止め　36
健康診断書　144
健康保険　5, 10
検査　26, 30
検査着　27
腱反射　23

こ
誤飲　133
抗凝固薬　36
抗菌薬　36
高血圧　20, 31
高コレステロール血症　31
抗ヒスタミン薬　36
誤嚥　133
国際結婚　2
国民健康保険　10, 12, 49
子育て　61
骨折　31
粉薬　44
コミュニケーション　3

さ
採血　27
寒気　16, 65
坐薬　35, 41
自己負担　49
自費　49

社会保険　10

し
手術　30
出産　20
昇圧薬　36
消炎鎮痛薬　35
紹介状　31
錠剤　36, 44
症状　16, 65
上部消化管造影検査　27
食後　35, 45, 46
食事の直前　35
食事療法　20
食前　46
食中毒　80
食物アレルギー　20, 115
食欲　16, 18, 54, 65
初診　11
食間　35
処方せん　47, 49
視力検査　27
シロップ　44
診察　22, 23
診察券　11, 13
診察台　23
新生児訪問　5
腎臓病　31
靱帯　31
診断　30
診断書　145
心電図　27
じんましん　118
診療明細書　49

すせそ
水剤　35
睡眠導入薬　35
睡眠薬　36
水薬　44
頭痛　16, 54, 65
生検　27
精神安定薬　36
精密検査　27
咳　54, 65
セ氏　14, 17
舌下薬　36
赤血球数　31
説明と同意書　146, 147
先天性甲状腺機能低下症　64
先天性心疾患　106
先天性副腎過形成症　64
先天代謝異常検査　5
総合感冒薬　35

たち
体温　77
多言語医療問診表　3
多言語生活情報　4
脱臼　27
打撲　127

156

知的障害　64
虫垂炎　31
超音波検査　27
聴力検査　27
鎮静薬　36

つてと
通院証明書　148
通園・登校許可書　152
つかまり立ち　59
つたい歩き　59
手足口病　88
手洗い　60
てんかん　104
点滴　33
糖尿病　20, 31, 121
突発性発疹　84
ドライシロップ　44
鈍痛　16

なに
内視鏡　131
内視鏡検査　27
内服薬　44
軟膏　36, 42
入院　30
入院証明書　149
入院診療計画書　150, 151
尿　14, 16
尿検査　27
尿失禁　16
尿路感染症　82
妊婦健診　5

ぬねの
塗り薬　43
熱　16
熱傷　130
熱性けいれん　55, 86
ねんざ　31
脳波　27

は
肺炎　21, 31, 74
肺炎球菌　56
歯痛　16
排尿　14
はいはい　59
吐き気　16, 18, 54, 65
発育障害　64
白血球数　31
発熱　14, 54, 65
鼻水　54
母親学級　5
歯みがき　60, 61
肥満　124

ひふ
ひきつけ　54, 65
ひとり歩き　59
フェニルケトン尿症　64
ヒブ　56
飛沫感染　70
百日咳　100
病歴　21
貧血　31
頻尿　16
風疹　55, 94
腹痛　16, 54, 65
プリックテスト　31
分娩証明書　154
分娩予定日証明書　153

へほ
ヘルパンギーナ　90
便　14
偏頭痛　16
便秘　14, 15, 16, 17, 54, 65
保険証　13
母子健康手帳　4, 5
発疹　20, 55, 65
母乳　62
ホモシスチン尿症　64
ポリオ　55

まみむめも
麻疹(はしか)　55, 92
麻酔　20
麻酔薬　36
末梢血酸素飽和度　31
水ぼうそう　55, 98
むくみ　54
メイプルシロップ尿症　64
目薬　42
モロー反射　57

ゆよ
輸血　20
養育医療　5
溶連菌感染症　72
予防接種　20, 21
予防接種証明書　140, 141, 142
予防接種の問診票　3
予防接種歴　140
予約　11, 47, 49

らりる
ライ症候群　71
リウマチ熱　72, 73
離乳食　62
離乳食の進め方の目安　63
利尿薬　36
良性　31
ロタウイルス　56

・本書の複製権・翻訳権・上映権・譲渡権・公衆送信権（送信可能化権を含む）は株式会社診断と治療社が保有します．
・JCOPY 〈㈳出版者著作権管理機構　委託出版物〉
本書の無断複写は著作権法上での例外を除き禁じられています．複写される場合は，そのつど事前に，㈳出版者著作権管理機構（電話 03-3513-6969，FAX 03-3513-6979，e-mail: info@jcopy.or.jp）の許諾を得てください．

小児科外来医療英語

ISBN978-4-7878-1834-8

2012 年 1 月 10 日　初版第 1 刷発行
2016 年 10 月 5 日　初版第 3 刷発行

編 集 者	中村安秀／中野貴司
発 行 者	藤実彰一
発 行 所	株式会社 診断と治療社
	〒100-0014　東京都千代田区永田町 2-14-2　山王グランドビル 4 階
	TEL　03-3580-2750（編集）　03-3580-2770（営業）
	FAX　03-3580-2776
	E-mail：hen@shindan.co.jp（編集）
	eigyobu@shindan.co.jp（営業）
	URL：http://www.shindan.co.jp/
	振替　00170-9-30203
表紙デザイン	株式会社ジェイアイ
イラスト	北川カズナ
印刷・製本	三報社印刷株式会社

Ⓒ Yasuhide NAKAMURA／Takashi NAKANO, 2012. Printed in Japan.　　　　［検印省略］
乱丁・落丁本はお取り替え致します．